Th Potbelly Syndrome

How Common Germs Cause Obesity, Diabetes, and Heart Disease

Russell Farris and Per Mårin, M.D., Ph.D.

Foreword by Richard P. Huemer, M.D.

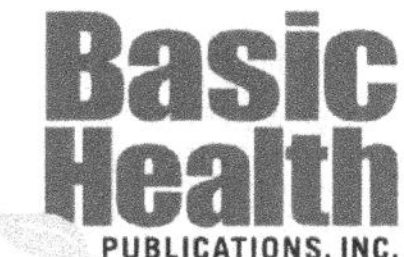

The information contained in this book is based upon the research and personal and professional experiences of the authors. It is not intended as a substitute for consulting with your physician or other healthcare provider. Any attempt to diagnose and treat an illness should be done under the direction of a healthcare professional.

The publisher does not advocate the use of any particular healthcare protocol but believes the information in this book should be available to the public. The publisher and authors are not responsible for any adverse effects or consequences resulting from the use of the suggestions, preparations, or procedures discussed in this book. Should the reader have any questions concerning the appropriateness of any procedures or preparation mentioned, the authors and the publisher strongly suggest consulting a professional healthcare advisor.

Basic Health Publications, Inc.
28812 Top of the World Drive
Laguna Beach, CA 92651
949-715-7327 • www.basichealthpub.com

Library of Congress Cataloging-in-Publication Data

Farris, Russell
The potbelly syndrome : how common germs cause obesity, diabetes, and heart disease / by Russell Farris and Per Marin ; foreword by Richard Huemer.
p. cm.
Includes index.
ISBN-13: 978-1-59120-058-1
ISBN-10: 1-59120-058-X
1. Chronic diseases—Etiology. 2. Obesity. 3. Diabetes. 4. Germ theory of disease. 5. Microorganisms. I. Marin, Per II. Title.

RB156.F37 2005
616.07'1—dc22

2005031713

Typesetting/Book design: Gary A. Rosenberg
Cover design: Mike Stromberg

Printed in the United States of America

10 9 8 7 6 5 4 3 2

Contents

To Norman Cousins
(1915–1990)

My determination is not to remain stubbornly with my ideas but I'll leave them and go over to others as soon as I am shown plausible reasons which I can grasp. This is the more true since I have no other purpose than to place the truth before my eyes so far as it is in my power to embrace it. . . .

—ANTONI VAN LEEUWENHOEK, THE FIRST GERM HUNTER, CIRCA 1700, QUOTED IN *MICROBE HUNTERS* BY PAUL DE KRUIF (1926)

Foreword

Potbellies have ever been with us, a fact of which I was reminded on a recent excursion to an art museum. I saw a depiction of William Penn's 1682 meeting at Shackamaxon with the Delaware Indians. There, on the left, were the Indians—bronzed, hale, well-proportioned; to the right of center was Penn, not yet forty, with his round face, spindly arms, and a prominent potbelly. Penn appeared cushingoid!—as well he might have been, given his stressful life: kicked out of college, imprisoned more than once in the Tower of London, and generally set upon for his antiestablishment views.

Cushing's syndrome often arises from stress, for stress goads the adrenal glands to produce cortisol, which is responsible for potbellies and other physical stigmata of Cushing's syndrome. Cortisol is also to blame for hidden, dark things like glucose intolerance and compromised immunity. In this book, Russ Farris and Dr. Per Mårin set forth lucidly the hypothesis that abdominal obesity, high blood pressure, excess fats in the blood, diabetes, and related ills share an underlying causative factor: chronic subtle hypercortisolism.

Dr. Mårin is a distinguished senior scientist, physician, and clinical teacher from Sweden, who has been writing on human obesity since 1985. Many of his eighty-two publications deal with the relation of hormones, including cortisol, to obesity. Russ Farris is not a doctor, but a retired artificial-intelligence researcher whose many years of service for the U.S. Navy included technical writing and editing. His ability to analyze the behavior of complex systems has served him well in assembling this book's big picture from many diverse elements of evidence.

Medical researchers like to break problems down into bite-size pieces, a process called reductionism. Thus, presented with a metaphorical elephant, one will describe the tail, another the legs, another the trunk, and so on. Each becomes an expert on his chosen piece of the puzzle. The authors of this book have put those pieces together, glimpsed the whole elephant, and named it the *potbelly syndrome.*

This is not your garden-variety health book, with self-assessment quizzes, menu plans, recipes, and nutritional supplement recommendations. There are, to be sure, many helpful suggestions about reducing stress, exercising, and taking care of medical conditions, along with a short list of supplements. Mainly, though, this is a book about asking why 47 million Americans suffer from a metabolic syndrome characterized by obesity, insulin resistance, high blood fats and sugar, and high blood pressure—and answering that question.

It is highly unlikely that Mr. Farris and Dr. Mårin will be flung into the Tower of London for their views, but their views are antiestablishment nonetheless. I expect acceptance of them initially to be an upstream swim against a tide of controversy, but honest dialogue is how medical science progresses, even in an era of managed care, rigid diagnostic codes, and governmental regulation. I wouldn't anticipate an outcome like that of a spawning salmon, whose upstream battle leaves it discolored, dysmorphic, and ultimately dead, suffused by a toxic concentration of its own cortisol.

Mr. Farris admits to having been influenced in his youth by Paul De Kruif's marvelous *Microbe Hunters,* as I was myself. It shows in his writing. As these pages unfold, enjoy Mr. Farris's clear and to-the-point prose style, along with the many diagrams for those who thirst for technical details. I know William Penn would have liked this book, not only because of his potbelly, but because of something he once said: "Speak properly, and in as few words as you can, but always plainly; for the end of speech is not ostentation, but to be understood." You will understand.

—Richard P. Huemer, M.D.

Acknowledgments

I'd like to thank my distinguished coauthor, Per Mårin, M.D., Ph.D., for his many contributions to this book. Dr. Mårin was an expert on the stress hormone cortisol for many years before I became interested in it. He gave me valuable suggestions, corrected many errors, tutored me on some of the finer points of endocrinology, and wrote the chapter on diagnosing chronic subtle hypercortisolism.

This book would not have been possible without the encouragement and sage advice of Bernard Rimland, Ph.D., Director of the Autism Research Institute. Dr. Rimland is my long-time friend and mentor, a philosopher of science without parallel, and the center of an amazing network of people who know interesting things. Dr. Rimland's friend Susan Owens provided the seed idea from which this book grew.

Woody McGinnis, M.D., and Sheldon Hendler, M.D., were the first physicians to hear my ideas on infections and cortisol. Donald Foster, M.D., was the first physician to read an early draft of the book. I was so unsure of myself when I started that a negative word from any of these gentlemen might have persuaded me to forget the book and go fishing. Instead, their encouragement and advice kept me going while I gained confidence.

Richard Huemer, M.D., reviewed drafts of the book and made suggestions that improved both its organization and its contents. Finding the answer to one of his questions probably delayed completion of this project by a year, but the book is much better for that delay. Dr. Huemer was gracious enough to write the foreword.

Allan Shor, M.D., described the circumstances that led him to discover *C. pneumoniae* in clogged arteries, and he gave me the amazing photograph shown in Figure 3.1.

My editor, Carol Rosenberg, made or suggested many improvements to the manuscript. I want to thank my publisher, Norman Goldfind, for recognizing the need for this book.

The Liz Fong Foundation provided encouragement and material support. I also received much help and good advice from the librarians at the University of California campuses in San Diego, Los Angeles, Irvine, Berkeley, and San Francisco.

More than a hundred people took the time to answer questions, give advice, send information, or help in other ways. I appreciate all of their input, but I particularly want to thank Emma Adam, M.D.; April Apperson-Farrell, M.S.; Burton Berkson, M.D.; Teresa Binstock; Alison Blake; J. Edwin Blaylock, M.D.; Robert Da Prato, M.D.; Elissa Epel, Ph.D.; Karin Everett, Ph.D.; Clara Felix; Diana Flory; Dr. Leigh Gibson; Kenneth Grattendick, Ph.D.; Ray Hanson; Les Hayes, Pharm.D.; Lane Heldfond; Robert Henry, M.D.; Abram Hoffer, M.D.; Denise Hooks; Dr. Gail Ironson; Dale Lieu, M.D.; Petru Liuba, M.D.; Sandra Marek; Martin Möckel, M.D.; Robert Munford, M.D.; Louise Pace; Dr. Laura Pawlow; Erkki Pesonen, M.D.; James Phillips, Ph.D.; Gerald Reaven, M.D.; Graham Rook, M.D.; Patty Schmidt; Mishi Sokolic; Charles Stratton, M.D.; Jennifer Tom; Brian Walker, M.D.; and David Wheldon, FRCPath.

Lastly, I want to thank my daughters, Letitia and Tamara, and my son Jay, for not complaining about promises not kept, trips not taken, and fish not caught while I worked on *The Potbelly Syndrome.*

—Russ Farris

Introduction

In the late eighties my doctor predicted that I (Farris) would die from a heart attack within ten years. I took him seriously, so I joined the long lines of dieters trudging to and from salad bars. I went to the gym more often, went for walks during lunch breaks, and took the stairs instead of elevators—still I grew fatter. After roughly ten years of fretting about my blood pressure, weight, and cholesterol, I had the predicted heart attack. I survived, but it was pretty clear that rabbit food and exercise were not working for me.

I had spent most of my life solving problems for the U.S. Navy, so I tried to view heart disease as just another interesting problem to solve. I began by browsing through several websites maintained by the U.S. National Institutes of Health (NIH), taking notes, and printing the abstracts of journal articles. After a few weeks, I saw that several lines of research were converging on a new explanation for heart disease. The following are its main features:

- We all have mild, chronic infections caused by common germs.
- Some of these germs produce sores in our arteries, just as other germs produce sores on our skin. The sores in our arteries are sometimes called lesions, plaques, atheromas, or atherosclerosis.
- Most heart disease is caused by sores growing in the arteries that supply blood to the heart.

My heart attack was not caused by eating too much or exercising too little—it was caused by germs living in my arteries. No amount of exercise and rabbit food would have killed those germs; therefore, no amount of exercise and rabbit food would have prevented my heart attack.

I used this new information about germs to my benefit, as I will explain in Chapter 1, and then I began to study obesity. My doctor, like most skinny people, was sure that anyone with enough willpower could lose weight and keep it off. I was finding that harder and harder to believe. I had enough willpower to go to college at night, work forty years, and teach a martial art. I had tons of willpower, but I never seemed to have enough to lose weight. There had to be a better explanation for my obesity, and I found it after a few months of research:

- Infections stimulate the production of a stress hormone called *cortisol.*
- Cortisol steals glucose (blood sugar) from our muscles and liver to make more glucose available to the brain.
- The brain seldom uses all of the extra glucose, so some of it is converted to visceral (abdominal) fat. When this happens frequently, we develop potbellies.

Cortisol robs our muscles and livers of glucose by a mechanism called insulin resistance (Chapter 8). Most doctors believe that obesity causes insulin resistance, but there is a lot of evidence that insulin resistance causes obesity. People with insulin resistance must eat extra food to compensate for the glucose stolen from their muscles and liver. Part of this extra food is converted to fat and deposited around our waist. Some people with insulin resistance are not overweight yet, but most overweight people are insulin resistant.

Advanced insulin resistance is often called Syndrome X or dysmetabolic syndrome X, but "potbelly syndrome" (PBS) is a more descriptive term. Type 2 diabetes is a very severe, long-term form of insulin resistance, and it is the last and worst stage of PBS. People with PBS usually have heart disease as well, but PBS and heart disease are separate conditions.

The Potbelly Syndrome dispels several myths about blood pressure, cholesterol, and dieting. For example, it is a myth that we can force our weight down and keep it down by limiting the amount of food we eat. Research shows that only one person in twenty, and perhaps only one person in a hundred, ever loses weight and keeps it off while dieting. In the long run, diets make us fat. Worse yet, even thinking about diets may make us fat (Chapter 12).

This book was written to help you avoid heart disease and PBS. If it's already too late to avoid these problems, this book can help you recover. The first few chapters explain how common germs cause heart disease and raise cortisol levels. Beginning with Chapter 6, the emphasis shifts toward cortisol-related illnesses: high blood pressure, obesity, and type 2 diabetes. *Chronic subtle hypercortisolism* is the technical term for potbelly syndrome, and Dr.

Mårin explains how to diagnose this disorder in Chapter 16. The remaining chapters offer suggestions for dealing with PBS and heart disease. Most chapters offer lists of suggested readings, and references are listed at the end of every chapter. There is a glossary near the end of the book in case you are unfamiliar with some of the medical terms used here.

To recover from heart disease and PBS, you will need the help of doctors who understand both germs and cortisol. There aren't many of these doctors yet, so you will have to help them a little for the next few years. At the end of each chapter is a reference list. We suggest that you give your doctors copies of any pertinent abstracts or articles mentioned in the reference lists. Most of the abstracts and many of the articles can be found on the Internet, but some are only available from medical libraries. Chapter 17 explains how to find scientific documents on the Internet.

Dr. Mårin and I hope that you will find this book both interesting and useful.

1

Germs and Potbellies

[The idea that germs cause chronic diseases] is so simple and so significant that one would think it would have been recognized by many and would be the starting point for any discussion of the causes of disease. Not yet.

—PAUL W. EWALD, *PLAGUE TIME*

When I (Farris) was twenty-two I worked at Cape Canaveral, and my work took me to South America and the Caribbean. On a trip to Brazil I became extremely ill, and while I was recovering I developed a large potbelly and several small, annoying health problems. I kept telling my doctors that I was infected with some rare tropical parasite, but they ignored me. After thirty-seven years of chronic illness, topped off by a heart attack, my health problems included:

- A huge potbelly that was still growing.
- Extremely high blood pressure.
- Migraine headaches, insomnia, fatigue, and depression.
- Feeling cold most of the time.
- Chronic sore throat, stuffy nose, and lung infections.
- Atrial fibrillations (rapid, erratic heartbeats).
- Irritable bowel syndrome.
- Chronic eye infections and deteriorating eyesight.
- Thin, dry skin with fungal infections, white scales, and dark blotches.

In February of 1999, I learned that I was infected with a bacterium that is now called *Chlamydophila pneumoniae* (CPN). CPN is not a rare tropical parasite; it is one of the most common germs on the planet. It affects some people more than others, and the older we get, the more likely we are to become infected with it.

I was given an antibiotic called clarithromycin, and within two months all of the illnesses listed above vanished. My potbelly was melting away. My heart was as steady as a metronome and my blood pressure dropped forty points. I found myself taking deep breaths just for the pleasure of feeling the air move freely in and out of my lungs. My legs seemed to have motors in them, and I walked for miles as easily as the wind blows. I felt like I was twenty years old again.

If I had stayed well, there wouldn't be any need for the rest of this book. You could jot "clarithromycin" on a scrap of paper and you would know everything you need to know about CPN and the diseases it causes. Unfortunately, I was back in the hospital with most of my old symptoms by July. CPN, it turned out, was not going to be so easy to get rid of.

Even though I was sick again, my outlook on life had improved one hundred percent between January and July. Feeling really good for the first time in decades, even if only for a few months, had shown me that a steady loss of health followed by an early death was not inevitable. One other thing became clear in those months—I could not depend on my HMO doctors to keep me well. If I was going to get well and stay that way, I would have to learn a lot more about my own health problems.

I had been haphazardly collecting materials for a book about CPN, but I didn't get serious until I saw that the beneficial effects of clarithromycin were wearing off. After that, I spent hundreds of hours reading abstracts from the United States government's PubMed database (www.ncbi.nih.gov/entrez/query.fcgi). If an abstract was particularly interesting, I would copy the entire article from the medical library on the San Diego campus of the University of California.

One day I stumbled onto an article about a chemical that made CPN grow faster in laboratory dishes. The chemical was *hydrocortisone succinate,* and it is a synthetic version of the stress hormone *cortisol.* Within a few hours of learning about hydrocortisone succinate and cortisol, I discovered that many of my health problems were identical to those of people with a cortisol-related disease called *Cushing's syndrome.*

CUSHING'S SYNDROME

In 1912, Harvey Cushing described one of his potbellied patients as follows:

> She has become stout, her weight increasing from 112 pounds two years ago to 137 pounds at present. Other noteworthy symptoms have been insomnia, tinnitus, extreme dryness of the skin, frequent sore throat, shortness of breath, palpitation, purpuric outbreaks, marked constipation, sudden attacks of dizziness with falling, a definite growth of hair and mustache during the last few years with marked falling out of the hair of the scalp. She feels chilly and cold all of the time and suffers from insomnia rather than from drowsiness. Muscular weakness is extreme and there is much complaint of backache and epigastric pains.[1]

This patient, Miss M.G., was only twenty-three years old. In addition to the disorders described above, she suffered from high blood pressure, headaches with nausea and vomiting, spontaneous nosebleeds, stunted growth, malformed bones, bleeding hemorrhoids, easy bruising, swelling of her feet, absence of menses, double vision, and bulging, painful eyes. Altogether, Miss M.G. had more than thirty separate disorders.

Miss. M.G.'s potbelly and all of her other ailments were caused by an excess of cortisol, a condition known as *Cushing's syndrome* or *hypercortisolism.* Miss. M.G.'s case was extreme, but millions of people have milder forms of hypercortisolism.

POTBELLY FACTS AND HYPOTHESES

At this point, from my experience with clarithromycin and my study of Cushing's syndrome, I knew three important facts about potbellies:

1. Potbellies are usually accompanied by some of the disorders Miss M.G. had.
2. Potbellies and potbelly-related disorders are often symptoms of hypercortisolism.
3. My potbelly shrank and my potbelly-related illnesses disappeared after taking a drug that killed bacteria.

From these facts, I developed three hypotheses:

1. Since I had many of the same disorders that Miss M.G. had, I might have hypercortisolism.

2. Since my cortisol-related problems disappeared after taking clarithromycin, it seemed likely that clarithromycin had somehow lowered my cortisol levels.
3. Since clarithromycin is best known for killing bacteria, maybe bacteria are able to raise cortisol levels.

My cortisol levels had not been measured yet, so there was no way to test my first and second hypotheses. My third hypothesis was confirmed by browsing through PubMed, where I learned that infections raise cortisol levels by initiating *acute phase responses* (Chapter 2). Acute phase responses (APRs) produce *inflammatory* substances to kill germs. Then they produce *anti-inflammatory* substances to protect us from the inflammatory ones. Cortisol is the most important anti-inflammatory substance.

Inflammatory substances and cortisol oppose each other, as shown in Figure 1.1, but together they manage to kill most germs and eliminate most inflammations. Some germs survive, however, producing mild inflammation and a small excess of cortisol for as long as we live. These are the germs that cause heart disease and potbelly syndrome.

POTBELLY SYNDROME

When we are young and have only a few chronic infections, cortisol does an excellent job of canceling the effects of inflammation. We look and feel good. Unfortunately, we accumulate more infections and inflammation as we get older. Our cortisol rises, but it does a poorer and poorer job of canceling the effects of inflammation. At the same time, the side effects of cortisol become stronger. We start to "feel our age."

The competing effects of inflammation and cortisol produce different results in everyone, but there are patterns of illness that recur in millions of people. One of these patterns is formed by the close association of abdominal obesity, high blood pressure, and high blood sugar. This pattern has had many names in recent years, including:

- Syndrome X
- Metabolic syndrome X
- Dysmetabolic syndrome X

All of the "X" syndromes are defined a little differently, and most researchers believe they are caused by poor diet or lack of exercise. Other

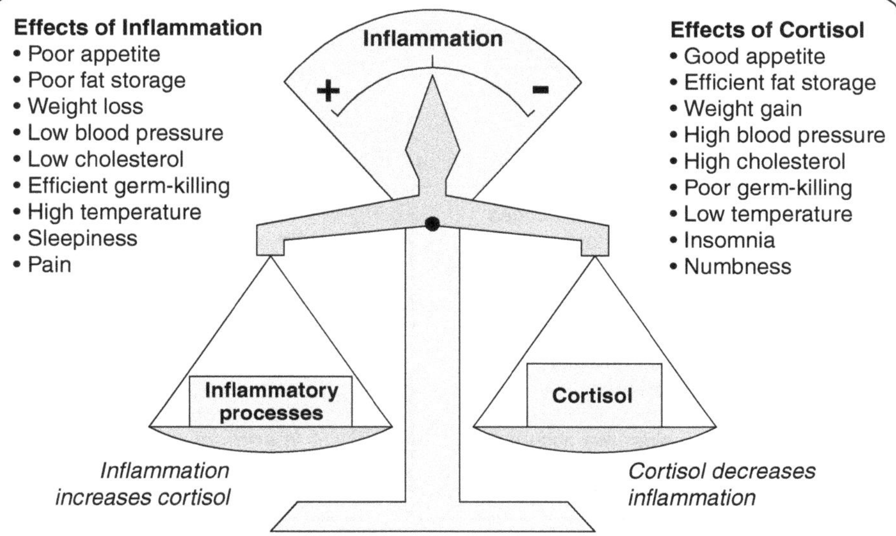

Figure 1.1. Inflammatory Processes and Cortisol Oppose Each Other
All adults have multiple chronic infections. If our particular combination of infections shifts the pointer toward the left side of the scale, we will lose weight and have more of the illnesses associated with inflammation.

If our infections are such that the pointer moves over toward the right side of the scale, we will gain weight and have more of the illnesses associated with cortisol. Most of us have a mix of both inflammatory and cortisol-related disorders.

researchers, who noticed that the X syndromes all resemble mild cases of Cushing's syndrome, suspect that they are caused by cortisol. Eventually, the arguments of this latter group convinced me that the X syndromes are in fact caused by cortisol. Since none of the existing X syndromes included cortisol in their definitions, I defined a new one, dropped the X, and called it *chronic subtle hypercortisolism.* That's an accurate term, but it is pretty awkward, so I call it potbelly syndrome or PBS for short. The main features of PBS are abdominal obesity, high blood pressure, and a small, long-term excess of cortisol. Type 2 diabetes is an extreme form of PBS. Dr. Mårin, who has studied cortisol and the X syndromes for many years, developed a more formal definition of chronic subtle hypercortisolism/PBS (Chapter 16).

Some of the same germs that cause PBS also cause heart disease. As shown in Figure 1.2, germs trigger acute phase responses that produce inflammation and cortisol. The inflammation causes heart disease, and the cortisol causes PBS. As you will see in later chapters, this theory fits the facts

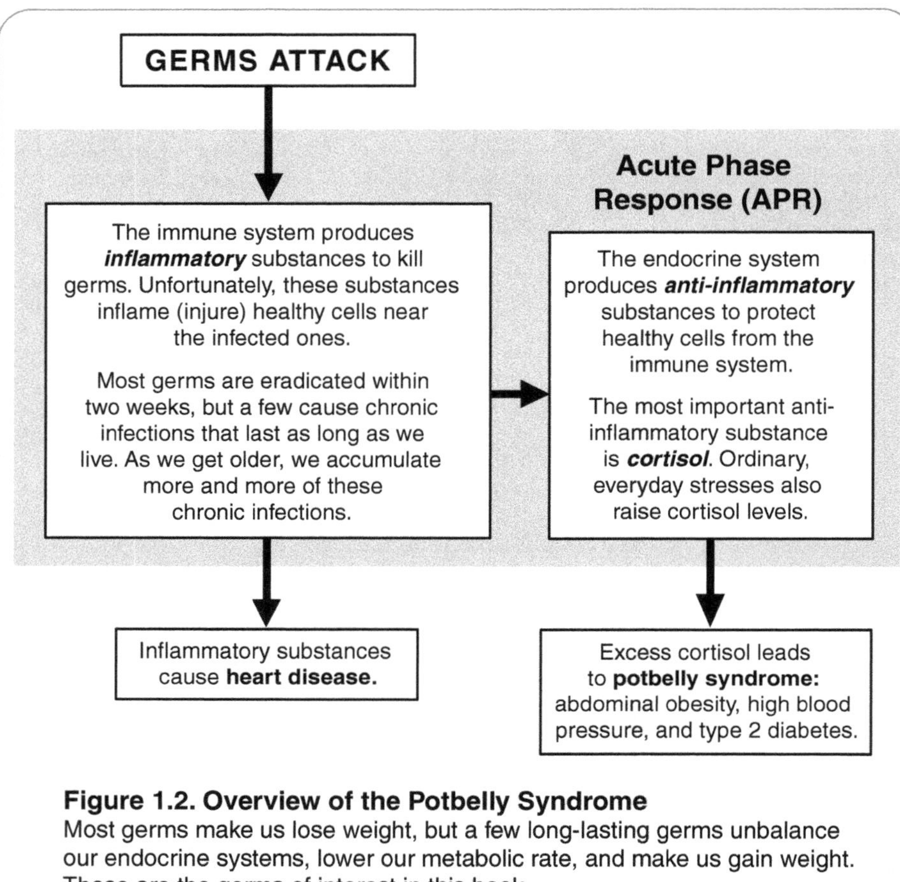

Figure 1.2. Overview of the Potbelly Syndrome
Most germs make us lose weight, but a few long-lasting germs unbalance our endocrine systems, lower our metabolic rate, and make us gain weight. Those are the germs of interest in this book.

pretty well, and it explains why diet and exercise cannot prevent either obesity or heart disease.

PBS AND HEART DISEASE ARE BOTH TREATABLE

My experience with clarithromycin was a little like finding the fountain of youth, then watching it go dry. Clarithromycin worked great, once, but the effects didn't last long, and it had less effect each time I used it. The same thing happened with other antibiotics, and my health deteriorated to the point where I knew which doctors worked each shift in my HMO's emergency room.

Many Kinds of Fat

Fat is stored in fat cells, and fat cells are grouped together in fat depots scattered around the body. *Subcutaneous* fat depots are located under the skin, where they provide insulation to protect us from cold. Subcutaneous fat is often called *diffused* fat.

Visceral fat depots are located around our *viscera* (internal organs). The viscera and the visceral fat are located in a sort of "bag" made from the abdominal muscles.

Abdominal fat is any fat between the chest and hips, and an excess of abdominal fat produces a potbelly. Visceral fat presses against the abdominal muscles and produces potbellies that are hard to the touch. Subcutaneous fat produces soft potbellies.

Researchers studying potbellies usually do not distinguish between visceral and subcutaneous obesity, so we will use the term *abdominal obesity* unless we are specifically referring to visceral or subcutaneous obesity.

Visceral fat accumulates in response to the hormone cortisol. The effect of cortisol on subcutaneous fat is not clearly established.

Between hospital visits, I worked on this book, and at some point I realized that I ought to focus on treatments more than causes if I wanted to be around to see the book in print. This insight prompted me to study ways to fight infections and reduce cortisol levels. What I learned has kept me pretty spry for several years, and some of it may help you. The best of the books I read are listed in the chapters where they will be of most interest, and the last four chapters are devoted to avoiding, or at least surviving, heart disease and potbellies.

SUMMARY

It's easy to see, now, why $170 worth of clarithromycin had such an amazing effect on my health. By killing at least some of my germs, clarithromycin lowered my cortisol levels. My potbelly and my potbelly-related illnesses faded away as my cortisol levels dropped. Clarithromycin could not kill enough germs to completely cure me, so I had a relapse a few months later. When the germs came back, my cortisol levels rose again and all of my cortisol-related illnesses returned.

Chronic infections, hypercortisolism, and PBS can be defeated, and learning about them is the first step toward victory. The next chapter explains how germs raise cortisol levels.

RECOMMENDED READING

At the end of most chapters, I have listed books and websites with additional information about infections or PBS-related topics. I don't agree with everything these books and websites say, but I think they are useful.

Microbe Hunters, by Paul de Kruif (Harvest Books, 2002).
This book is one of the all-time classics in medical literature. It begins with the first microbe hunter, Antoni van Leeuwenhoek, and it ends with Paul Ehrlich's attempts to cure syphilis in the 1920s. For some unknown reason there was a copy of Microbe Hunters *in our barn when I was a kid, and it was one of the first books I read.*

New Guinea Tapeworms and Jewish Grandmothers, by Robert S. Desowitz (American Museum of Natural History, 1981).
Germs that make us fat won't seem half as strange after you read Dr. Desowitz's funny and fascinating book. In fact, I recommend reading all of his books.

Parasite Rex, by Carl Zimmer (Free Press, 2001).
The host-parasite interactions described in Parasite Rex *are creepier than the movie* Alien. *The pictures are astonishing.*

Plague Time, by Paul W. Ewald (Free Press, 2000).
This book describes the unending battle between humans and germs. It is beautifully written and easy to understand. It does not discuss the germ-cortisol interaction, but it describes many of the other tricks germs use to attack us.

REFERENCES

Epigraph: Ewald, Paul W. *Plague Time: How Stealth Infections Cause Cancer, Heart Disease, and Other Deadly Ailments.* New York, NY: Free Press, 2000, p. 56.

1. Cushing, Harvey. *The Pituitary Body and Its Disorders: Clinical States Produced by Disorders of the* Hypophysis Cerebri. J.B. Lippincott Company, 1912, p. 217.

2

Stress, Infections, and Cortisol

Cortisol . . . belongs to a class of hormones called glucocorticoids, which affect almost every organ and tissue in the body. Scientists think that cortisol has possibly hundreds of effects in the body.

—EILEEN CORRIGAN, NATIONAL INSTITUTES HEALTH

Our adrenal glands produce three important stress hormones: epinephrine (adrenaline), norepinephrine (noradrenaline), and cortisol. Epinephrine and norepinephrine are the famous "fight or flight" hormones that prepare us for instant action. They are only produced in response to fairly large stressors, and they usually don't have much effect on our general health. Cortisol, however, is always present in the bloodstream, so small changes in stress produce corresponding changes in cortisol levels.

Cortisol is so powerful that a slight excess can—over a period of years—have terrible effects on our health. We will discuss those effects in later chapters; here we will focus on the small stresses that cause most cases of potbelly syndrome.

STRESSES, STRESSORS, AND STRESS RESPONSES

Technically, *stresses* are changes caused by *stressors*. When you climb stairs, your foot pressing down on a step is a stressor; the slight downward bending of the step is a stress. This simple terminology is complicated by the fact that many stresses are also stressors. In the following chain of stressors and stresses, each item is a stressor to the items listed below it and a stress caused by the thing above it:

- A cold wind blows across bare skin (unequivocally a stressor).

- Blood vessels constrict to reduce the flow of blood to the skin and preserve the warmth of the body. (Blood vessel constriction can be called either a stress or a stressor, depending upon the context in which it is being discussed.)
- Blood pressure rises (unequivocally a stress in this example).

The general public never adopted the word *stressor*, so *stress*, *stressed*, and *stressful* are usually applied equally to stresses and stressors. To make it easier to recognize causes and effects, many writers now use the expression *stress response* (or *stress reaction*) instead of *stress* to indicate a change caused by a stressor. In this book we will use:

- *Stressor* when speaking of something that causes a stress response.
- *Stress response* when speaking of something that was caused by a stressor.
- *Stress* when it doesn't matter whether we are speaking about a stressor, a stress response, or both (this is usually the case).

Good stress and bad stress. Stress researchers sometimes divide stress into two categories: *eustress*, which makes us stronger, healthier, or happier, and *distress*, which does the opposite. When we use the term *stress* in this book, we are usually speaking of *distress*.

STRESS RESPONSES

There are thousands of stressors that can annoy, frighten, or injure us enough to trigger stress responses, but we have only a small number of physiological responses that we can make to each stressor. One of those responses—and the most frequent—is the production of stress hormones.

The *hypothalamus* determines whether to release stress hormones. It is an ancient, primitive part of the brain, and it responds to a honking car horn the same way it would respond to a snarling mountain lion—it triggers the release of stress hormones. Philip Gold, from the U.S. National Institute of Mental Health, describes stress responses this way:

> . . . The stress response is an evolutionary response to danger: a system that prepares us to fight or flee. Our bodies produce stress hormones such as cortisol, epinephrine, and norepinephrine that affect us by breaking down certain tissues to mobilize fuel, increasing our heart rate, preparing our muscles to move us. All these responses are necessary when we are in dan-

ger, but they can have long-term medical consequences if stress becomes our chronic state.[1]

Once the stress hormones are released, our bodies and minds are changed in ways that will help us to survive simple, short-term stressors. These changes are so similar, regardless of the stressor, that they are sometimes referred to as *stereotypical* (or *generalized*) stress responses. Most of the stereotypical stress responses are produced by cortisol, most are helpful in the short term, and most are harmful in the long term. Table 2.1 lists some of our stereotypical responses to stressors.[2]

TABLE 2.1. COMMON RESPONSES TO STRESSORS

Response to Stressors	Cortisol Causes Response	The Response: Helps Us Short Term	The Response: Harms Us Long Term
RESPONSE OF HYPOTHALAMUS			
Triggers release of cortisol and other stress hormones		■	■
METABOLIC RESPONSES (POTBELLY SYNDROME)			
Increased cholesterol in blood	■	■	■
Increased blood pressure	■	■	■
Accumulation of fat	■	■	■
Increased appetite (in chronic stress)	■	■	■
Increased sugar (glucose) in blood	■	■	■
Increased thirst and urination	■		
OTHER PHYSIOLOGICAL RESPONSES			
Weakened immune system	■	■	■
Impotence	■		■
Loss of appetite (in acute stress)		■	■
Nervousness and tensing of muscles		■	■
COGNITIVE RESPONSES			
Increased alertness, hypervigilance	■	■	■
Decreased attention and concentration		■	■
Tendency to oversimplify problems		■	■
Reduced creativity, imagination		■	■

Response to Stressors	Cortisol Causes Response	The Response: Helps Us Short Term	Harms Us Long Term
BEHAVIORAL RESPONSES			
Tendency to overeat	■	■	■
Less time spent sleeping	■	■	■
Less movement (saves energy)	■	■	■
More likely to be violent		■	■
More likely to break rules		■	■
Tendency to use alcohol and drugs			■
EMOTIONAL RESPONSES			
Anxiety, irritability, hostility	■	■	■
Reduced interest in sex	■	■	■
Depression	■		■
Less interest in being with others		■	■
Less self-esteem			■
Hopelessness, poor motivation			■

Note that every stress response listed in Table 2.1 is, in its extreme form, a serious mental or physical illness. We cannot cover all of these disorders in this book, but we will discuss stress-related metabolic problems in detail (Chapters 5–13).

When we get an infection, the immune system initiates an *acute phase response* (APR) to kill the germs. APRs are stressful, so they trigger the release of stress hormones. The extra stress hormones, in turn, produce some of the stereotypical responses listed in Table 2.1. The next few pages will explain how infections cause APRs and how APRs raise cortisol levels.

FLU-LIKE SYMPTOMS

Have you ever wondered why infections as different as AIDS, Ebola, and the common cold always start with a runny nose and a fever? The reason is that no matter what kind of germ it is that attacks the body, our immune system initiates an acute phase response (APR). APRs are all very much alike, and it is the APR, not the germ, that causes the early symptoms. The peculiarities that distinguish one infection from another develop later.

APRs start in recognizable stages, but each stage continues to operate after the next one begins. Consequently, the stages overlap each other throughout most of the APR.

Stage 1. Immune System Activation

Cells "talk" to one another by releasing chemical messengers called *cytokines.* About a hundred cytokines have been discovered, but we have no idea what most of them do. Some of them appear to carry "help me!" messages, and some seem to carry "I'm okay, leave me alone" messages.

In the earliest stage of an APR, infected cells release "help me!" cytokines to activate the immune system. The immune system consists mainly of immune cells—the white blood cells you learned about in high school—plus the lymph nodes scattered throughout the body. While lymph nodes are important to our health, they aren't important to our discussion of APRs, so we won't discuss them here.

As "help me!" cytokines from infected cells drift through the blood, some of them bump into immune cells. The cytokines tell the immune cells to move toward the infected cells.

When the immune cells reach the infected cells, they "read" the cytokines and decide what to do. If the invading germs are outside of the cells, the immune cells try to kill the germs and eat them. If the germs are inside the cells, the immune cells kill the infected cells and then eat the dead cells and any germs that remain in them. In either case, the chemicals used by the immune cells are very toxic and injure nearby cells. The injured cells are said to be *inflamed*.

Stage 2. Cytokine Cascade

Germs try to overwhelm the immune system by reproducing and spreading quickly. To prevent them from taking over the whole body, the immune system produces huge armies of immune cells and sends them to the infected areas. Consequently, germs and immune cells race to out-reproduce each other. To help the immune cells win this race, inflamed cells join the infected cells in secreting "help me!" cytokines to attract more immune cells. As new immune cells arrive, they release still more cytokines to attract still more immune cells, and the inflammation spreads rapidly from cell to cell. This produces a snowball effect known as a *cytokine cascade.*

Cytokine cascades do a great job of killing germs, but they cause fevers, sore throats, muscle aches, malaise (feeling "awful"), headaches, sleepiness, and generally give us those notorious "flu-like symptoms."[3] They also ruin our appetites, reduce our ability to store fat, lower our blood pressure, and raise our body temperature.

Since "help me!" cytokines are at the heart of this inflammatory process, they will be referred to as *inflammatory* cytokines from now on. The inflammatory cytokines of greatest interest to people with potbellies are *interleukin-1* (IL-1), *interleukin-6* (IL-6), and *tumor necrosis factor-alpha* (TNF-alpha). These are sometimes called the *primary cytokines,* and their appearance is an important link in the chain of events that leads from infections to potbellies.

Stage 3. Liver Activation

The bloodstream carries cytokines to every part of the body. When inflammatory cytokines reach the liver, they trigger the release of *acute phase proteins* (APPs). APPs are not very well understood, but it appears that some of them try to reduce the damage done to cells by cytokine cascades. Other APPs may kill germs directly or indirectly.

One of the primary cytokines, IL-6, stimulates the production of an APP called *C-reactive protein* (CRP). Even though we don't know what CRP does, many researchers believe that it is the best single indicator of the amount of inflammation present in the body. Consequently, your CRP level can give your doctor valuable information about your health.

Stage 4. Controlling Cytokine Cascades

To reach their target tissues and organs, cytokines, immune cells, and germ-killing chemicals have to circulate through the bloodstream. Because of this, an infection anywhere in the body spreads inflammatory substances throughout the body. If nothing stops it, a cytokine cascade that starts in a big toe can grow until it becomes a *cytokine storm* that inflames every cell in the body. Cytokine storms kill people in about three days.

Fortunately, the primary cytokines—IL-1, IL-6, and TNF-alpha—all stimulate the production of cortisol, and cortisol prevents cytokine cascades from becoming cytokine storms.

Fortunately, the primary cytokines—IL-1, IL-6, and TNF-alpha—all stimulate the production of cortisol, and cortisol prevents cytokine cascades from becoming cytokine storms.

The immune system is made up of several subsystems, and cortisol inhibits the subsystems that cause cytokine cascades. This reduces the activity of immune cells, and it reduces the production of germ-killing chemicals. Consequently, our immune cells are not able to kill as many germs as they did when cortisol levels were lower. In other words, cortisol weakens the immune system to save us from potential cytokine storms.

Stage 5. Resolution

Up to this point, all infections are very similar, but from here on they follow one of three different paths:

- **Acute nonfatal path**—This is the most common case. The immune system quickly eradicates the new germ and our cytokine, APP, and cortisol levels return to normal. This is the path taken by common infections such as mumps and measles.
- **Chronic-acute (middle) path**—Sooner or later, we all encounter middle-path germs like *Chlamydophila pneumoniae.* We can't kill them and they can't kill us, so we carry them to the grave (or perhaps it is more accurate to say that *they* carry *us* to the grave). While we live, our bodies are flooded with extra cytokines, APPs, and cortisol.
- **Acute fatal path**—This is the least likely path. Germs that kill us quickly, such as the Ebola virus, are scary but they do not infect many people.

In this book, we are only interested in middle-path germs, the slow-acting germs that stay with us for life unless we, with the help of our doctors, make intense efforts to kill them. The effects of these middle-path germs are additive, so each one makes us a little sicker than the one before it.

Figure 2.1 summarizes the main features of the acute phase response. You don't need to memorize the details, but you might want to dog-ear the page so you can refer to it when we discuss APRs in later chapters.

THE BENEFITS OF CORTISOL DO NOT COME CHEAPLY

Once or twice every year we get the sniffles and maybe a little fever. We assume that we have a cold, or maybe the flu, and we expect it to go away in a few days. We take some extra vitamin C and forget about it. In most cases, the germ was harmless and the immune system eradicated it. Occasionally, maybe once every three or four years, we get roughly the same symptoms,

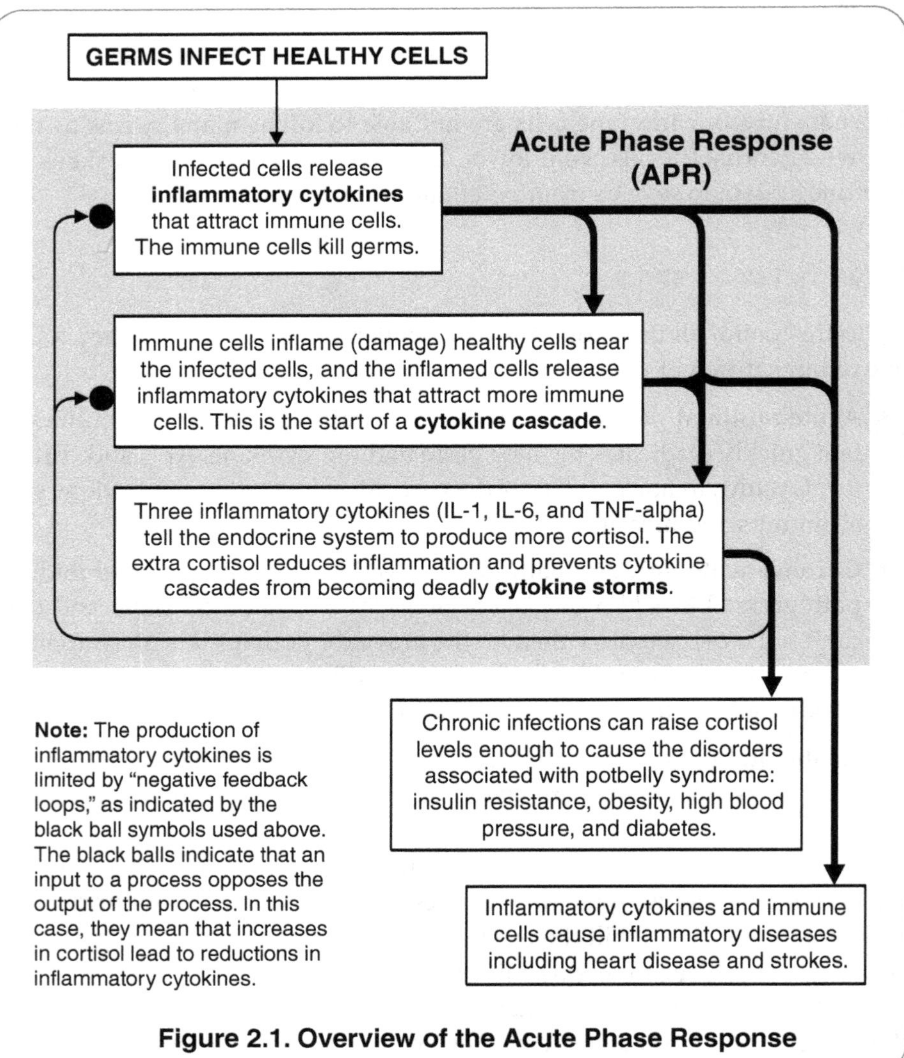

Figure 2.1. Overview of the Acute Phase Response

but they last longer. We can't quite kill this new germ, so we learn to live with it—we adapt. From then on, the immune system produces a few more cytokines and immune cells than it did before, the liver produces more acute phase proteins, and the endocrine system produces more cortisol. We almost never know that we have made these adaptations.

These adaptations are part of Mother Nature's plan to keep us alive and active during our child-bearing and child-rearing years. If we are sick or injured, cortisol lowers our temperature, raises our blood sugar, numbs our pain, and keeps us awake so we can work and take care of our children. At the same time that cortisol is keeping us up and working, it is suppressing our immune system and allowing germs to grow in our arteries, joints, and nerves. It is also disrupting our metabolism in ways that will lead to obesity and diabetes for many of us.

The aches and pains of old age are, to a large extent, part of the high price we pay for the benefits we received from cortisol when we were young.

SUMMARY

Infections flood our bodies with immune cells, cytokines, acute phase proteins, and cortisol. These substances keep us alive and functioning, but they make us gain weight and feel lousy. The more infections we have, and the longer we have them, the worse we look and feel. Some chronic infections are curable, but curing them requires a deliberate effort by you and your doctor.

RECOMMENDED READING AND RESOURCES

The books and websites listed below provide information on lowering stress levels and boosting our immune systems.

NIH websites: *An excellent way to learn more about infections and the immune system is to check out the tutorials available on various NIH websites. I particularly recommend the one provided by the National Cancer Institute at* www.cancer.gov/cancertopics/understandingcancer/immunesystem.

Thorn in the Starfish: The Immune System and How It Works, by Robert S. Desowitz (W.W. Norton, 1988).

This book is a joy to read. It is worth a trip to the library just to read Chapter 9: "Eating Your Way to Immunity."

The U.S. Army War College Guide To Executive Health and Fitness, edited by William F. Barko and Mark A. Vaitkus (August 2000).

This online book contains a lot of clearly written information on stress and cortisol. It can be downloaded from www.cdc.gov/nccdphp/dnpa/usphs/pdfs/army.pdf

Why We Get Sick, by Randolph M. Nesse, M.D., and George C. Williams, Ph.D. (Random House, 1994).

This book presents illness from an evolutionary perspective. Medical professionals and science buffs will find it fascinating.

REFERENCES

Epigraph: NIH Publication No. 90-3054. February 12, 1998.

1. Gold, PW. "The High Costs of Stress." U.S. National Institute of Mental Health. www.loc.gov/loc/brain/emotion/Gold.html.

2. *Some of the material in this section was adapted from: Aeromedical Training: Stress Defined.* Office of the Adjutant General, 1st Battalion (GSAB) 140th Aviation Regiment. February 3, 2004.

3. Beisel, WR. Herman Award Lecture, 1995: Infection-Induced Malnutrition—from Cholera to Cytokines. *Am J Clin Nutr* 1995 Oct;62(4):813–819.

3

Germs That Cause Chronic Illnesses

. . . in the past two decades, dozens of pathogens have been implicated in a range of diseases, from Alzheimer's to arthritis. Recently, some biologists have argued that evolutionary theory predicts that all but the rarest chronic diseases must be caused by infections.

—CARL ZIMMER, *SCIENCE*, SEPTEMBER 14, 2001

Middle-path germs are common, but they are not well known, so we will look at a few of them before I show you, in later chapters, how they cause heart disease and potbelly syndrome.

CHLAMYDOPHILA (CHLAMYDIA) PNEUMONIAE (CPN)

CPN is probably the most important middle-path germ. It infects between 40 and 70 percent of all adults in the United States, and it has been linked to more than forty diseases and conditions, including:

- Alzheimer's disease
- Arthritis
- Asthma
- Atherosclerosis
- Bronchitis
- Chronic obstructive pulmonary disease (COPD)
- Diabetes
- Earache
- Encephalitis
- Endocarditis
- Follicular conjunctivitis
- Giant cell arteritis
- Hepatitis
- Hypertension
- Immune suppression
- Interstitial cystitis
- Iritis
- Kidney failure
- Lung cancer
- Meningitis
- Multiple sclerosis
- Myocarditis
- Obesity
- Pericarditis
- Pharyngitis
- Pneumonia
- Porphyria (secondary)
- Prostate cancer
- Prostatic hyperplasia
- Prostatitis
- Sinusitis
- Syndrome X
- Vasculitis

CPN is linked to many diseases, but it is not the *sole* cause of any known disease. Consequently, you could have several of the diseases listed above and still not be infected with CPN. But then again, you might be, and if you are infected with CPN you can expect to develop more problems as you get older and your immune system weakens.

Life History of CPN

CPN is so common that we are exposed to it every day, and almost everyone who can be infected is already infected. Men are more susceptible than women, and old people are more susceptible than young ones. People with other infections, such as herpes viruses, are more susceptible than healthy people.

CPN is spread by coughing. Our bronchial airways are lined with hair-like cilia that wiggle continuously to move mucus up and out of our lungs. CPN paralyzes the cilia so that the only way to clear our airways is to cough—if we don't cough, we drown. When an infected person coughs, he or she fills the air with a fine mist of bronchial fluids containing CPN. If a susceptible person inhales that mist, he or she will be infected.

CPN infections usually start in the tissues that line the nose and breathing passages, then spread to the lungs. Victims develop the "flulike symptoms" that we discussed in Chapter 2. At the same time, immune cells called *macrophages* become infected. Macrophages don't travel much, so the infection may not move past the lungs for a long time. Eventually, however, the infection spreads to immune cells called *monocytes.*

Monocytes drift through the bloodstream to every part of the body. After about two weeks they stop drifting, burrow into our flesh, and turn into macrophages. Monocytes that are infected with CPN turn into infected macrophages. Macrophages can live for several months, and when they die the CPN organisms inside of them may either escape and infect nearby cells or continue to live inside the dead macrophage. If an infected macrophage is eaten by another immune cell, that immune cell may become infected too. Thus some of our immune cells, the cells that protect us from most germs, keep themselves and us infected with CPN year after year.

This cycle of infection goes on throughout the body, but it is particularly intense in the smooth muscles in our arteries. Figure 3.1 shows part of a smooth muscle cell crammed full of CPN. The small, dark organisms are sporelike *elementary bodies* (EBs). They are so small that they are just a fuzzy blur on a conventional microscope (the photograph in Figure 3.1 was made

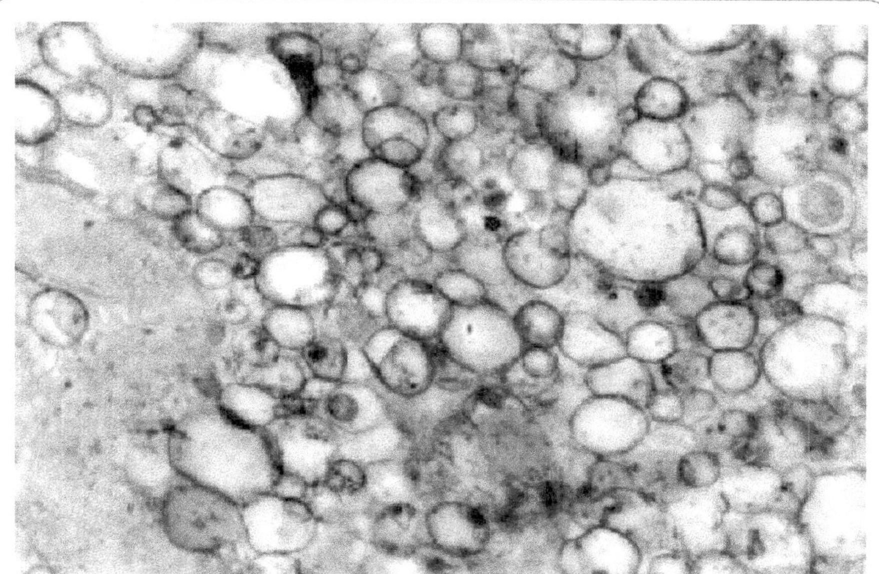

Electronmicrograph courtesy of Dr. Allan Shor, National Centre for Occupational Health, South Africa.

Figure 3.1. CPN Organisms Filling a Human Smooth Muscle Cell
The smaller, darker organisms are spore-like *elementary bodies* (EBs). They are biologically inactive until they get inside of a host cell that has been weakened by cortisol, injury, or old age. When conditions are right, EBs turn into potato-shaped *reticulate bodies* (RBs) and begin to reproduce. When the host cell is stuffed with RBs, as in this photo, the RBs change back into EBs. When the cell dies, the EBs are released to infect other cells. EBs are extremely difficult to kill.

with an electron microscope). Hard to see and hard to kill, EBs can live for up to thirty hours on a tabletop. If a susceptible person touches a contaminated surface and then touches her nose, eyes, or mouth, she is likely to become infected.

When an EB touches the side of a cell, the cell mysteriously opens up and pulls the EB inside. The EB tries to disable the cell's germ-killing systems. If it is successful, it turns into a larger, potato-shaped *reticulate body* (RB) and begins to reproduce. If an invading EB cannot immediately turn off a host cell's germ-killing system, it waits until the cell is weakened by damage, cortisol, or age and then it turns into an RB.

RBs steal energy from the cell and reproduce at a furious pace. When a cell is crammed full of RBs, the RBs turn into *intermediate bodies* (IBs), and the IBs quickly turn into new EBs. The EBs dissolve the wall of their host cell and

CPN's Old Name

CPN's official name was *Chlamydia pneumoniae* for several years, and many scientists still use the old name, including the authors of the treatment protocols discussed on pages 26–27. CPN is not the same germ as the sexually-transmitted *Chlamydia trachomatis*.

escape into the space between cells and start the cycle all over again. The entire cycle, from EB to RB to IB to new EB, can occur in as little as seventeen hours, or it may take months, depending upon the strength of the germ-killing systems in each cell.

Treatment of CPN Infections

In 1999, it was widely believed that clarithromycin would cure CPN infections, and for a few months I thought I had been cured. Unfortunately, no single drug will eradicate CPN. Our immune cells protect the EBs from antibiotics, so reinfection begins as soon as any single-drug treatment ends.

Through a stroke of luck, I learned about a CPN patient in Hawaii who was being treated with multiple drugs in an antichlamydial protocol developed by Charles Stratton and William Mitchell, two researchers from Vanderbilt University. Dr. Stratton shared the protocol with my doctor, who gave it to me. Dr. Stratton stressed that the protocol was experimental, and that it was being sent for humanitarian reasons. He asked us not to disseminate it widely.

At the time, I estimated that it would cost less than a $1,000 to implement the protocol's recommendations, but my HMO doctors would not cooperate because they thought the recommendations were "too experimental." Ironically, my giant HMO has spent tens of thousands of dollars on me since then to treat my CPN-related illnesses.

Even though I have not had any help from my HMO, I have used the Stratton-Mitchell protocol as the foundation of my fight to stay well. I believe the fact that I am alive and writing today is due in part to following—as much as possible—the advice given by Drs. Stratton and Mitchell.

An updated version of the protocol has been patented, so I am released from my promise of silence. Unfortunately, the four or five pages of practical advice contained in the new protocol are mixed in with a hundred pages of legal and medical jargon. If you feel up to the challenge of making sense out of the patent, you can download it from the Internet by going to the U.S. Patent and Trademark Office's website (http://patft.uspto.gov/netahtml/srchnum.htm) and searching for patent number 6,579,854.

Fortunately, there is an easier way to get help in fighting CPN. Dr. Stratton has been working with Dr. David Wheldon, a British medical microbiologist. Dr. Wheldon has an anti-CPN protocol on his website that has many of the same features as the earlier Stratton and Mitchell protocols. This new protocol was designed for people with multiple sclerosis, so parts of it may not be applicable to other people with CPN infections. The protocol is available from www.davidwheldon.co.uk/ms-treatment.html. A one-page summary of the protocol is available from www.davidwheldon.co.uk/cpn-treatment.pdf. A list of supplements recommended by Dr. Wheldon is provided in Chapter 19 of this book.

Will these protocols cure CPN infections? No one knows yet because the protocols are still experimental. The only thing we know for sure about treating CPN in the year 2005 is that there is no single drug that will eradicate all three forms of the germ. I have benefited from these protocols, but I want to make it very clear that they were not designed to be home remedies. Eradicating a CPN infection will require a long, intensive effort by you and your doctor.

CYTOMEGALOVIRUS (CMV)

Cytomegalovirus (CMV) is a herpes virus that infects half of all people over age thirty, and nearly everyone over age sixty. It usually doesn't present any symptoms, but it may cause blindness and a mononucleosis-like illness. CMV causes pneumonia in people with impaired immune systems, and it kills many organ-transplant recipients. CMV is a cortisol-loving germ; in a laboratory study where human cells were grown in dishes and then infected with CMV, adding cortisol to the dishes increased CMV's ability to infect human cells eleven-fold.[1]

CMV and CPN are often found together, and they are linked to many of the same diseases. Like CPN, CMV infects immune cells and suppresses the immune system.[2]

GERMS THAT CAUSE GUM DISEASE (PERIODONTITIS)

The germs that cause gum disease are suspected of causing heart disease and type 2 diabetes. Gum disease occurs with greater frequency and severity among people with diabetes, and it has been assumed for years that the diabetes caused the gum disease.[3] There is some evidence, however, that it is the other way around. Researchers from Buffalo, New York, used an antibiotic to treat the infected gums of type 2 diabetics. As expected, the patients' gum health improved. More interestingly, the patients' hemoglobin A1c levels dropped 10 percent.[4] (Hemoglobin A1c levels are indicators of the severity of a patient's diabetes.)

This was a small test, and a 10 percent drop in hemoglobin A1c levels is not very spectacular, but it suggests that the antibiotic was killing germs that were contributing to the patients' diabetes. Would a more aggressive treatment with different antibiotics bring about larger improvements in the health of diabetics? No one knows—this was the only study of its kind.

HUMAN PAPILLOMA VIRUS (HPV) AND SKIN TAGS

Most of the information in this book came from long hours of searching through the PubMed website and digging through the stacks of the University of California–San Diego medical library. The most interesting items, however, were often discovered by accident, and such is the case with skin tags. Bernard Rimland, Ph.D., Director of the Autism Research Institute, gave me an article by Jonathon Wright that mentioned Syndrome X, a condition that resembles PBS. The article also contained an interesting anecdote about researchers who found that 80 percent of their patients with skin tags either had diabetes or developed it within five years.[5] I was never able to track down all of the details of Dr. Wright's story, but I found a few studies in PubMed that linked skin tags to diabetes, insulin resistance, and body-mass index (BMI).[6,7]

Skin tags (achrochordons) are small sacks of skin that grow on the neck, armpits, and groin. They are harmless, but they are often removed for aesthetic reasons. The most interesting fact about skin tags is that they are caused by the human papilloma virus (HPV)—the same virus that causes cervical and vulvar cancers.

THE INFECTION-CORTISOL LOOP

At this point, a reasonable question might be: "I can see how a germ might kill me quickly, before my immune system has a chance to adapt to it, but how can germs like CMV and CPN dodge my immune system year after year?" The answer to this question requires a short side trip into the theory of evolution.

I am a big fan of Richard Dawkins, a British evolutionary biologist. In *The Selfish Gene,* Dr. Dawkins describes how living creatures adapt to the pressures and opportunities that exist in their environments. Any Dawkins fan who stumbled onto the twin facts that (1) infections raise cortisol levels and (2) cortisol suppresses the immune system would guess instantly that germs were exploiting cortisol for their own benefit. A few hours of browsing through PubMed were enough to learn how they do it:

1. All germs trigger acute phase responses (APRs).
2. APRs produce inflammation, which tends to kill germs.
3. Inflammations trigger the release of cortisol, and cortisol tends to protect germs.
4. During APRs, some germs—we will call them X germs because some of them cause "X" syndromes like PBS—are helped more by the extra cortisol than they are hurt by the inflammation.
5. X germs that raise cortisol levels a lot survive better, and become more numerous, than X germs that do not raise cortisol as much.
6. Return to step 1.

Infection-cortisol loops like this one have been operating in mammals for millions of years, and the X germs that infect us now are very good at raising cortisol levels. The middle-path germs that cause obesity, high blood pressure, type 2 diabetes, and heart disease are all X germs. The germ that causes AIDS is also an X germ, and its interaction with cortisol was first described in a 1986 paper written by Robert Da Prato and Jonathon Rothschild:

> A state of chronic relative cortisol excess. . . . inhibits successful anti-pathogen strategies including those directed against the AIDS virus itself and leads to a self-sustaining downhill clinical course.[8]

Although Drs. Da Prato and Rothschild focused on the virus that causes AIDS, their paper made it clear that other germs could initiate and sustain similar loops. NIH researchers George Chrousos and Philip Gold developed their own version of the infection-cortisol loop. It was described as follows in a news release from the NIH:

> In response to an infection, or an inflammatory disorder like rheumatoid arthritis, cells of the immune system produce three substances that cause

> inflammation: interleukin-1 (IL-1), interleukin-6 (IL-6), and tumor necrosis factor (TNF). These substances, working either singly or in combination with each other, cause the release of . . . cortisol. Cortisol and other compounds then suppress the release of IL-1, IL-6, and TNF, in the process switching off the inflammatory response.
>
> Ideally, stress hormones damp down an immune response that has run its course. When [we are under continual stress,] that damping down can have a down side, leading to decreased ability to release the interleukins and fight infection.
>
> In addition, the high cortisol levels resulting from prolonged stress could serve to make the body more susceptible to disease, by switching off disease-fighting white blood cells.[9]

Infection-cortisol loops are operating inside of each one of us right now, and middle-path germs are raising our cortisol levels and suppressing our immune systems. They are also making some of us obese and diabetic, and they are destroying the arteries of some of us. The last four chapters discuss methods of slowing down, and perhaps blocking, infection-cortisol loops.

WHY WE GET MORE INFECTIONS AS WE GET OLDER

Infection-cortisol loops grow in strength with every new infection. When we get a new infection, our cortisol rises a little and all of our old germs benefit. They grow a little stronger, and in doing so they weaken the immune system still more. The additional weakening of the immune system then makes us more susceptible to new germs, which further weaken us. Figure 3.2 shows how all of this happens. The net result of this cooperation by germs is that we acquire new infections at an accelerating rate as we get older. Furthermore, the effects of our infections become worse with age.

If you want to learn more about the effects of multiple infections, visit the PubMed website and review the recent work of Hans-Jürgen Rupprecht and his associates. Dr. Rupprecht never mentions cortisol, but his research shows that the effects of infections are cumulative.

MERCIFUL GERMS?

Since infection-cortisol loops weaken our immune system so much, you may be asking: "Why don't new infections kill us in a few days?" Sometimes they do. Millions of people in poor countries die of runaway infections, and every year thousands of Americans die from strep and pneumonia despite the best

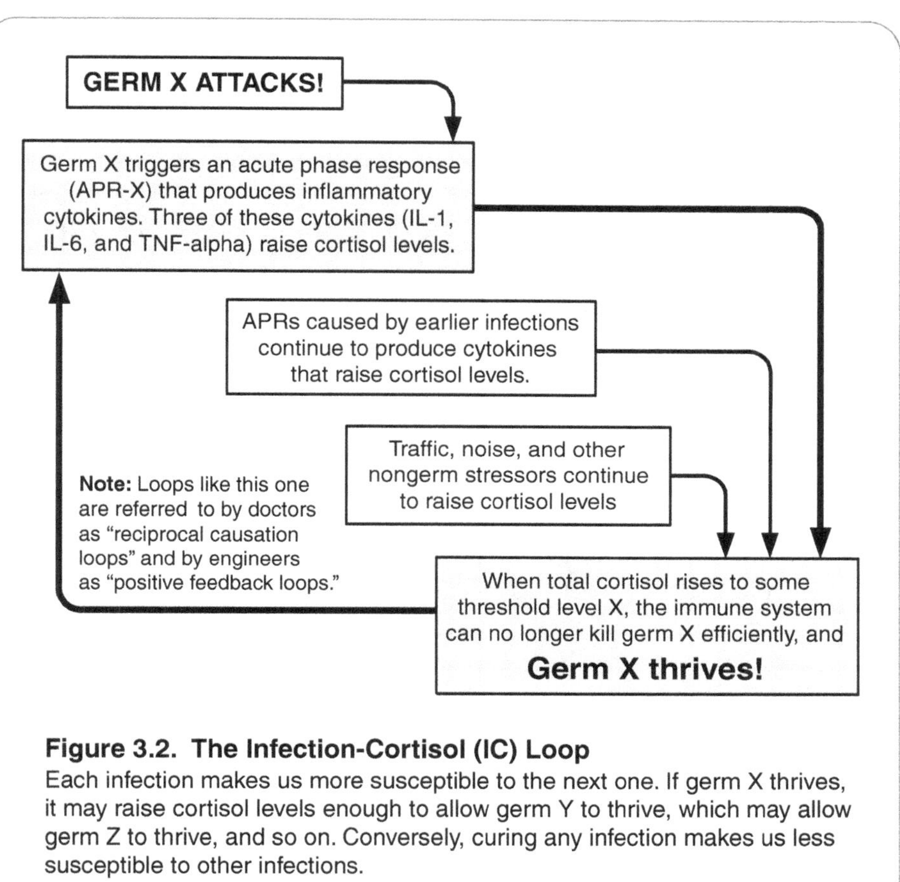

Figure 3.2. The Infection-Cortisol (IC) Loop
Each infection makes us more susceptible to the next one. If germ X thrives, it may raise cortisol levels enough to allow germ Y to thrive, which may allow germ Z to thrive, and so on. Conversely, curing any infection makes us less susceptible to other infections.

efforts of modern medicine. Most of us survive, however, because the germs want us to.

Germs want us to stay alive so that we can feed them and provide them with warm, moist homes. They want us to hug and kiss our loved ones, shake hands with our friends, and sneeze on strangers. Germs want us to drive them to PTA meetings and Little League games where they can meet new people. They want us, in short, to be their slaves. The diseases they cause are accidents—collateral damage, to put it in military terms.

To keep us infected but still breathing, the most successful germs have learned to maintain a happy balance (happy, at least, for them). They do this by raising our cortisol levels high enough to weaken us, but not high enough to kill us right away.

DIAGNOSING CHRONIC INFECTIONS

If you are infected with several middle-path germs, you probably don't feel great, but you may not feel awful either. Most of the time you just feel kind of blah. It's the kind of feeling that makes you want another piece of lemon pie even though you're not hungry. It's the kind of feeling that makes you want to sit down and watch TV instead of taking your grandkids fishing. It is not an acute illness and it's not health; it is the middle path described in Chapter 2. Family doctors are not trained to look for middle-path germs, so the most important step in learning which germs are making their homes in us is to find an expert who understands them.

Infectious disease specialists are more likely than other doctors to be experts on chronic infections, and you can get their names from the American Medical Association (AMA). The AMA lists most of the doctors in the United States, and you can find infectious disease specialists in your area by going to http://dbapps.ama-assn.org/aps/amahg.htm. Click on "Search for a Physician" and follow the instructions on each web page. I did this and got a list of thirty-five infectious disease specialists in or near San Diego, California. A "specialist" is not necessarily an expert, but the AMA website is a good place to start looking for an expert.

If you are old enough to have grandchildren, you are probably infected with CPN, CMV, or both. Identifying your other infections can be tricky. Since it is not practical to test you for every germ on the planet, your doctor has to make educated guesses about the germs that are likely to be living in you. Your doctor needs to be a good guesser because there are about 140 germs that frequently cause human illnesses.

The most common tests are called *serology* tests, and they measure chemicals (antibodies) produced by your immune system. Since middle-path germs have been fooling your immune system for years, the chemicals produced by your immune system do not provide a very good basis for diagnosis. Consequently, serology tests are not very accurate. They're cheap, though, so it is a good idea to have them—just don't take them too seriously. If the results of a serology test are positive for germ X, then it is pretty certain that you are infected with germ X. If test results are borderline, you should consider them positive until an infectious diseases specialist tells you otherwise.

If you are being diagnosed at a large institution, and money is no object, your doctor may order polymerase chain reaction (PCR) tests like the ones portrayed on *CSI* and other television shows. PCR tests can often find CPN in our monocytes even when serology tests indicate that we are not infected.

It is difficult to diagnose chronic infections by their symptoms. Since immune systems vary from person to person, the germs that survive and the symptoms they cause will also vary. In one person, CPN can survive in the lungs but not in the arteries. In the next person, the reverse may be true. CPN is best known as a cause of pneumonia, yet it causes only 10 percent of all cases. Similarly, CPN causes heart attacks in some people, but thousands of people without a trace of CPN still have heart attacks.

Have yourself tested for CMV, CPN, and any other germs your doctor recommends if any of the following circumstances apply to you:

- You are a smoker.
- You have chronic respiratory or sinus infections.
- You have any heart problems.
- You are over fifty years old.
- You have several of the conditions listed at the beginning of Chapter 1.
- You have several of the CPN-related conditions listed on page 23.

A C-reactive protein (CRP) test will tell you how much inflammation there is in your body at any given time. Since infections are a major source of inflammation, a high level of CRP suggests that you have serious infections. It can't tell you what is causing the infections, however. CRP tests currently cost about thirty dollars.

WHAT TO DO ABOUT CHRONIC INFECTIONS

A few pages back we saw that germs cooperate with each other, and every new germ makes us more susceptible to still more new ones. Conversely, eradicating any germ weakens all of our other germs. Once your doctor knows what middle-path germs you are carrying, she may be able to kill some of them, and thereby weaken the others.

Unless the protocols discussed on pages 26–27 work, we have to assume that CPN infections are incurable at this time. Still, antibiotics can clear them up for a few months, and during those months, your body can repair itself to some extent. Also, a few months of feeling good can do wonders for your spirits.

If you have any of the supposedly harmless viral infections such as CMV or herpes simplex, check with your doctor to learn how to keep them from flaring up. Your doctor will probably tell you to minimize the amount of stress in your life, a topic that will be discussed in Chapter 18.

SUMMARY

Common germs seldom cause life-threatening illnesses in healthy people, but many of them, like the ones discussed in this chapter, raise our cortisol levels. Since excess cortisol causes PBS, it isn't surprising that all of the germs discussed in this chapter are linked to one or more of the PBS disorders (obesity, high blood pressure, and type 2 diabetes).

Each infection weakens our immune system and makes us more susceptible to the others. The damage they do is additive, and the more infections we have, the worse we look and feel.

Diagnosing and treating chronic infections is difficult because they are usually caused by intracellular germs that hide in our own cells. You can't expect your family doctor to know much about these germs—you need help from infectious disease specialists, and more particularly, you need help from doctors who are experts in chronic infections.

RECOMMENDED READING AND RESOURCES

Diagnosis and Management of Infection Caused by Chlamydia, by William M. Mitchell and Charles W. Stratton. U.S. Patent number 6,579,854.

The Natural Guide to Beating the Supergerms and Other Infections Including Colds, Flus, Ear Infections, and Even HIV, by Richard P. Huemer, M.D., and Jack Challem (Pocket Books, 1997).
This is the best of the do-it-yourself books dealing with the immune system. My copy has dozens of dog-eared pages.

The Selfish Gene, second revised edition, by Richard Dawkins (Oxford University Press, 1990).
Dawkins proposes a thought experiment in which we imagine that living organisms are the vehicles that genes use to reproduce more genes. When we look at infection, predation, and war from the viewpoint of genes, many of the mysteries of life are a little less mysterious.

The Ten Best Tools to Boost Your Immune System, by Elinor Levy, Ph.D., and Tom Monte (Houghton Mifflin, 1997).
This is an excellent book full of practical advice on diet, vitamins, and stress reduction. I think the authors are wrong about saturated fat, and I think that they get cause and effect backward at times, but I still recommend this book.

REFERENCES

1. Koment RW. Restriction to human cytomegalovirus replication in vitro removed by physiological levels of cortisol. *J Med Virol* 1989 Jan;27(1):44–47.

2. Jones TR, Hanson LK, Sun L, et al. Multiple independent loci within the human cytomegalovirus unique short region down-regulate expression of major histocompatibility complex class I heavy chains. *J Virol* 1995;69:4830–4841.

3. National Diabetes Information Clearinghouse. 1999 Mar. *Diabetes Statistics in the United States.* NIH Publication No. 99-3926.

4. Grossi SG, Skrepcinski FB, DeCaro T, et al. Treatment of periodontal disease in diabetics reduces glycated hemoglobin. *J Periodontol* 1997 Aug;68(8): 713–719.

5. Detect and prevent diabetes NOW—years, even decades in advance! *Nutrition & Healing.* 2001 July; 8(7).

6. Casanova-Romero PY, Florez HJ, and Goldberg RB. Acanthosis nigricans and achrochordons in insulin resistant subjects with and without glucose intolerance: A study in three ethnic groups. *DIEAEAZ* 1999; 48(1): A167–168.

7. Hollister DS and Brodell RT. Finger "pebbles." A dermatologic sign of diabetes mellitus. *Postgrad Med* 2000 Mar;107(3):209–210.

8. Da Prato RA and Rothschild J. The AIDS virus as an opportunistic organism inducing a state of chronic relative cortisol excess: Therapeutic implications. *Med Hypotheses* 1986 Nov;21(3):253–266.

9. Stress System Malfunction Could Lead to Serious, Life Threatening Disease. News release from the U.S. National Institutes of Health, Monday, September 9, 2002.

4

How Germs Cause Atherosclerosis

Atherosclerosis, the major cause of coronary heart disease, begins during early childhood. . . . Humans experience, from early childhood, repeated acute infections. Chronic infections commonly undergo, within the same individual, repeated relapses accompanied by acute inflammatory and autoimmune reactions. These processes appear to be key-factors in the pathogenesis of atherosclerosis. . . .

—PETRU LIUBA ET AL., *EUROPEAN HEART JOURNAL*, 2003

Magazine ads produced by drug and food manufacturers give the impression that atherosclerosis is caused by little pieces of cholesterol drifting through the bloodstream looking for an artery to clog. The truth is both more complicated and more interesting.

BOILS, LESIONS, AND ARTERIAL PLAQUES

When I was a boy I had boils every summer, and, being a science nerd, I learned as much about them as I could. I found out that boils develop when hair follicles become infected with staph germs. The germs are quickly attacked by immune cells that crawl into the infected follicle (this, of course, is the acute phase response discussed in Chapter 2).

The immune cells eventually kill the germs, but many of the immune cells die, too. The dead germs and immune cells form a core of cream-colored pus inside of the follicle. If the core of the boil is near the surface, the cap of skin covering it pops open and the pus oozes out. If the core is deep, the pus may be enclosed in scar tissue, and the scar tissue and pus will make a bump that lasts for years.

Lesion is a technical term that doctors use for boils and other kinds of sores, and *lesion* is one of the names that doctors give to sores that develop in our arteries. Another name is *atheroma,* a Latin word that means "a tumor full of pus."[1] The injured area containing the lesions/atheromas is called *plaque.* That's right—the famous arterial plaques we hear so much about are just areas of scar tissue and pus. When we have a lot of pus in our arteries, we have *atherosclerosis.*

HEALTHY ARTERIES

Before we discuss diseased arteries any further, let's take a minute to study a healthy one. Figure 4.1 shows the most important layers of an artery. The outermost layer, the *tunica externa,* is made up of fine, tough fibers that run every which way to make a fabric that is soft and flexible, but strong enough to keep the artery from expanding too much under pressure. The middle layer, the *tunica media,* is made of smooth muscles that are wrapped around the innermost layer, the *tunica intima.* By contracting or relaxing, the smooth muscles can control the amount of blood flowing through the artery.

The inner layer is made of flat, delicate *endothelial* cells. They act like filters to control which substances from the blood go to which cells. In a healthy artery, blood never touches the smooth muscle cells in the middle layer.

The three layers of an artery should be very distinct—there should never be any smooth muscles in the inner or outer layers, and there shouldn't be any endothelial cells in the middle layer. Now we can return to our discussion of diseased arteries.

THE STAGES OF ATHEROSCLEROSIS

Germs have been attacking us, and our ancestors before us, for millions of years. Our war with germs continues, but we have managed to establish truces with middle-path germs like CMV and CPN. In return for giving them food, warmth, and transportation, middle-path germs let us live long enough to bear and raise our children. After that, the truce ends and they begin to kill us off in large numbers. Some middle-path germs live in our arteries, and the damage they do can be divided into three overlapping stages.

Stages of Atherosclerosis	Approximate Age
1. Initiation	Birth to 15 years
2. Progression (acceleration) stage	10 to 50 years
3. Complications (destabilization) stage	50 or more years

The ages given above are for typical cases, but damage to our arteries can be initiated at any age, and complications such as strokes and heart attacks often occur long before we reach fifty. Each stage is described on the following pages.

Initiation (First Stage)

Atherosclerosis begins with an injury to an artery. The injury could be from a cut or a bruise, but most injuries are caused by infections. Regardless of the

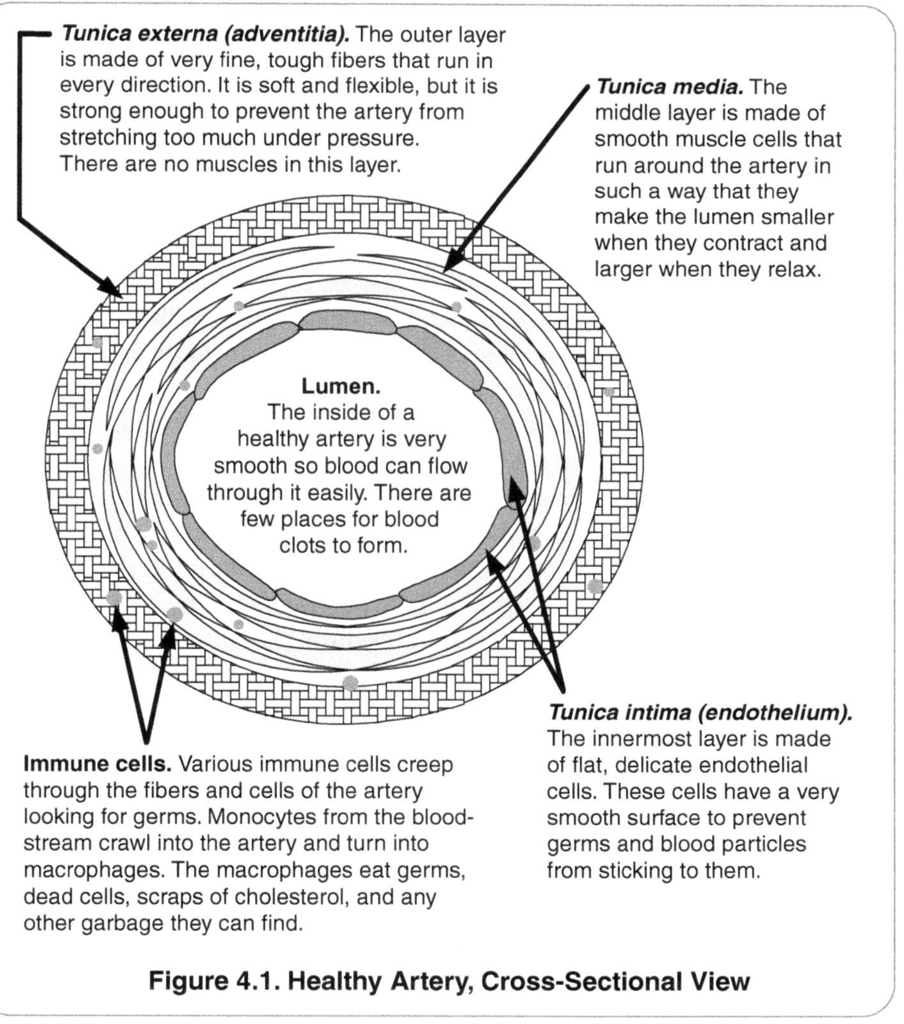

Figure 4.1. Healthy Artery, Cross-Sectional View

cause, each injury triggers an acute phase response and the artery becomes inflamed. The inflamed cells release cytokines that attract immune cells, and millions of germs and immune cells die in or near the inflamed tissue.

In a boil, the dead germs and immune cells are squeezed into a hair follicle and form a round core of pus about the size of a grain of rice. In an artery, the pus is squeezed between the layers of the artery so that it makes yellowish streaks. These streaks are sometimes found in the arteries of infants and they are common in teenagers. If a pregnant woman has a serious infection, her child may be born with atherosclerotic streaks. In other words, the earliest stage of atherosclerosis begins in infancy or childhood, long before we become obese.

Pus is very inflammatory, so the streaks may continue to attract immune cells and grow long after the original infection disappears.

Progression (Second Stage)

In stage two of atherosclerosis, scar tissue and smooth muscles form a cap over the streaks of pus, but the streaks continue to grow as more immune cells crawl into the artery and die. The smooth muscle cells, which are normally confined to the middle layer of the artery, begin to grow helter-skelter into the inner and outer layers. The flat endothelial cells that line the inside of the artery are killed, although some of them just move from the inner layer to the middle layer. The flexible strands in the outer layer are replaced with scar tissue. Over a period of several years, the artery becomes a complete mess, like the one shown in Figure 4.2.

Some of the damage done to the artery is caused directly by the invading germs, but a lot of it is done by the acute phase response that is trying to kill the germs. This isn't as bad as it sounds—the germs might kill us in days or weeks, but acute phase responses may take fifty years to finish us off. Still, it would be better if the acute phase responses didn't kill us at all.

The streaks get larger and larger until they merge together to form large cores of pus. The pus presses against the cap, and the cap expands out into the *lumina* (opening) of the artery as shown in Figure 4.3. Eventually the pus and the cap reduce the size of the lumina enough to restrict blood flow.

The narrowing of the lumina is called *stenosis,* and the restricted blood flow is called *ischemia.* If the ischemia is severe, it prevents our muscles and organs from getting enough oxygen, and this condition is called *hypoxia.* Hypoxia causes chest pain (angina), and severe hypoxia is deadly. Arterial lesions grow slowly, so we may have stenosis and ischemia for years before we develop hypoxia.

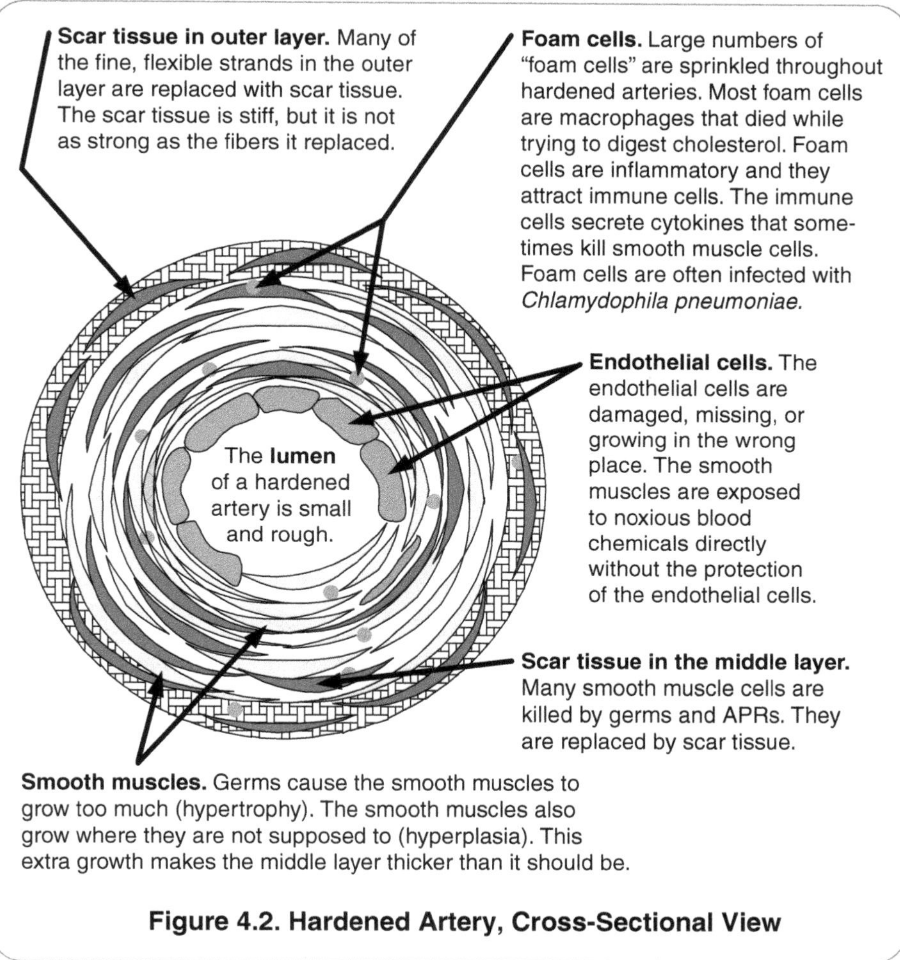

Figure 4.2. Hardened Artery, Cross-Sectional View

Although they are alike in many ways, there are some differences between boils and atherosclerotic lesions. Boils, for example, are always caused by staph germs, but the lesions in our arteries can be caused by many germs, including:

- *Chlamydophila pneumoniae* (CPN), my personal *bête noire.*
- *Helicobacter pylori,* a bacterium that causes ulcers and stomach cancer.
- The germs that cause gum disease.
- Herpes viruses, especially cytomegalovirus.

Since boils and plaques are caused by different kinds of germs, they involve different kinds of immune cells and have different kinds of pus. Most of the pus in a boil comes from immune cells called neutrophils, but most of the pus in a plaque comes from immune cells called macrophages. Neutrophils are mostly protein, but macrophages are mostly fat—to be more specific, the dead macrophages found in arterial plaques are full of cholesterol.

Macrophages are the garbage collectors of the body, and they creep through our flesh searching for germs, dead tissues, and dead immune cells to eat. They also eat small scraps of cholesterol that are left over from various bodily processes. Normally, macrophages process the cholesterol, excrete it, and go on with their garbage-disposal activities. The liver disposes of the processed cholesterol.

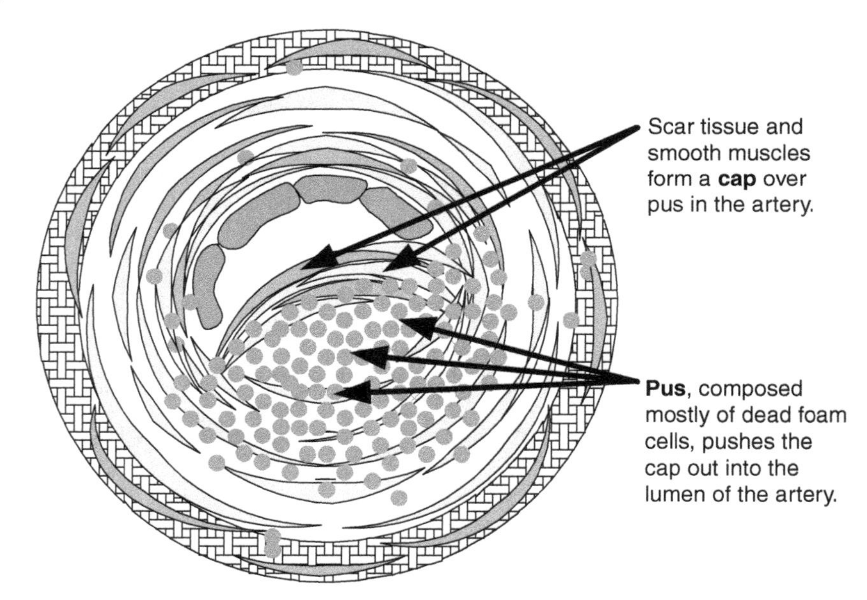

Figure 4.3. Artery Clogged By an Atheroma, Cross-Sectional View
An atheroma in an artery is similar to a boil. There is a cap made of smooth muscles and scar tissue. Pus pushes the cap out into the artery where it obstructs the flow of blood. The caps are not very strong, and pus oozes into the bloodstream when a cap breaks.

Caps have rough surfaces, so blood clots tend to form on them. If a coronary artery is blocked by a blood clot or a blob of pus, a heart attack occurs. If a cerebral artery is blocked, a stroke occurs.

In people with atherosclerosis, macrophages have trouble processing cholesterol and they never excrete it. Consequently, they gradually swell up and turn into *foam cells*. Foam cells tend to die in clumps, and these cholesterol-rich clumps form the streaks and cores of pus found in atherosclerotic plaques.

Complications (Third Stage)

The opening in the center of an atherosclerotic artery is small, and plaques are very "sticky," so blood cells called platelets sometimes clump together at plaques and form blood clots. These clots often cause heart attacks and strokes. Aspirin and other blood-thinning drugs are used to reduce the stickiness of platelets.

Plaques are classified as either stable or unstable, and stable plaques may exist in our arteries for decades without causing any trouble. Occasionally, for reasons that are not well understood, plaques become unstable. When this happens, the cap covering a core pops open and pus oozes into the bloodstream. The pus is carried into smaller and smaller arteries until it either breaks up or blocks an artery. If the pus blocks a coronary artery, we have a heart attack; if it blocks a cerebral artery, we have a stroke.

THE LINK BETWEEN CPN AND ATHEROSCLEROSIS

In the 1880s, germs were the hottest things in medicine, and many researchers assumed that atherosclerosis was caused by germs. Unfortunately, the germs that cause atherosclerosis are too small to be seen clearly with conventional light microscopes, so heart disease researchers eventually lost interest in germs.

A century later, Allan Shor, a pathologist working for the South African National Centre for Occupational Health (NCOH), was one of the thousands of people trying to discover the cause of atherosclerosis. Dr. Shor had spent hundreds of hours peering into light microscopes examining small sections of atherosclerotic tissue, seeing the same things that had been seen by thousands of researchers before him. Then, in 1990, NCOH obtained an electron microscope. With it, Dr. Shor saw the same things that he had seen before, but now he saw them more clearly. Small blobs that were barely detectable with the best light microscopes were now seen to have distinctive shapes and features. At first, Dr. Shor assumed, like everyone before him, that the blobs were droplets of fat. There is a lot of fat in atherosclerotic lesions, and these blobs weren't all that interesting to look at. Most of them resembled lumpy white potatoes. In the following excerpt from a 1999 letter, Dr. Shor describes what happened after several months of examining these blobs:

> After looking at hundreds of sections to no avail, it suddenly occurred to me that some of the structures we were looking at were not fat droplets at all, but more likely, small microorganisms or viruses of some kind. (The usual story of finding something new, of seeing what everyone had seen, but thinking what nobody had thought.)[2]

Dr. Shor and his colleagues spent six months trying to identify the potato-shaped microorganisms—the germs—he had discovered. They tried to grow the germs in their laboratory without success. After measuring every detail of the germs, Dr. Shor and his colleagues decided that the germs they were finding in plaques were similar to a germ called TWAR.

It was an example of either extraordinary good luck or great detective work to suspect that Dr. Shor's potato-shaped blobs were TWAR organisms. TWAR was not a well known germ in 1990. It had been discovered in 1965 and then forgotten for many years. In 1983, the same year in which the AIDS virus was discovered, TWAR was rediscovered in the lungs of students at the University of Washington in Seattle. The rediscovery of TWAR went unnoticed by most of the medical world, and by 1990 only sixty-five papers had been written about it. By comparison, more than 40,000 research papers were written about AIDS during the same period.

Researchers from the University of Washington had been authors or coauthors of nearly half of the papers written about TWAR, so Dr. Shor sent pictures and sample tissues to professor Cho-Chou Kuo at the University of Washington. Dr. Kuo confirmed Dr. Shor's suspicion that the potato-shaped germs were TWAR—the germ we now call *Chlamydophila pneumoniae* or CPN. The discovery of TWAR/CPN in atherosclerotic arteries generated tremendous excitement in the handful of people who knew about it in 1991.

In early 1991, Dr. Shor wrote a paper describing how he and his colleagues had found CPN (TWAR) in diseased arteries. He submitted it to a medical journal, but the editor decided not to publish it. A few months later, Dr. Shor presented a similar paper at a medical conference in South Africa. The paper was well received, and within the next year hundreds of researchers became interested in CPN. Since then, more than 800 articles have been published by researchers studying the links between CPN and atherosclerosis. Researchers have found CPN in almost every organ and tissue in the human body, and it has been found in dogs, horses, koalas, and frogs.

Dr. Shor's discovery prompted medical researchers to look for other germs in atherosclerotic plaques. Several were found, with most of the attention being focused on *cytomegalovirus* (CMV). This research has been complicated by the fact that people infected with CMV are likely to be coinfected with CPN.

Soon after CPN was discovered in atherosclerotic arteries, researchers began to suspect that it might be responsible for the formation of foam cells. To test this theory, researchers from the University of Wisconsin grew macrophages in the presence of CPN and cholesterol. They found, as expected, that CPN caused macrophages to turn into foam cells.[3]

Many Names for One Small Germ

To help you learn more about CPN via the Internet, I have summarized the convoluted sequence of names used for CPN since it was first discovered. Here are the names, in chronological order:

- TW-183 was the name given to CPN when it was discovered in the eye of a Taiwanese child in 1965.
- AR-39 (acute respiratory agent 39) was the name given to CPN after it was discovered in the lungs of University of Washington students in 1983.
- TWAR and TWAR-183 are acronyms formed from earlier names.
- *Chlamydia* TWAR is a name used occasionally after 1983. It is almost never used now.
- *Chlamydia pneumoniae* was the official name of CPN from 1989 to 1999.
- *Chlamydophila pneumoniae* has been the official name of CPN since 1999.

CPN's name has changed so many times that some researchers are sticking to the earlier name, *Chlamydia pneumoniae*, despite the fact that CPN is very different from its cousins in the *Chlamydia* genus. CPN is related to *Chlamydia trachomatis*, the sexually transmitted chlamydia, but it is not the same germ.

The name *Chlamydophila pneumoniae* is slowly gaining acceptance. When doing Internet searches, you will get the most hits by searching for *Chlamydia pneumoniae*, but you will get newer information by searching for *Chlamydophila pneumoniae*.

MEDICAL NEWS CAN TRAVEL VERY SLOWLY

In 1998, I was lying in a hospital room with tubes running in and out of my nose and arm. I had enough wires on me to hook up a jumbo set of Christmas tree lights. One morning my dapper young cardiologist came striding into my room to tell me that I'd had a heart attack. I had kind of guessed that, but I didn't want to hurt his feelings by mentioning it. As he was leaving, I asked him if my heart attack could have been caused by *Chlamydia pneumoniae* (CPN). He gave me a condescending smile and told me that *Chlamydia* might make me sterile, but it wouldn't cause a heart attack.

I was flabbergasted. At that time, hundreds of articles had been published about *C. pneumoniae,* and this ignorant pup didn't know the difference between *C. pneumoniae* and the sexually transmitted *C. trachomatis.* I got another cardiologist as soon as I could.

Later I learned that medical news travels swiftly from laboratories to the pages of medical journals, but it often takes years for news to reach practicing doctors. Perhaps I was expecting too much of my young cardiologist in 1998.

Seven years later, most physicians know the difference between *C. pneumoniae* and *C. trachomatis,* but that doesn't mean they believe that germs cause heart disease. When a doctor is forced to accept that atherosclerosis is caused by germs, not fat, then that doctor must learn a lot of new ideas and unlearn a lot of old ones. Doctors aren't any fonder of this learning/unlearning process than you or I would be, so many of them are downplaying the role of germs in heart disease. When it became clear a few years ago that most plaques contained germs of one kind or another, many doctors argued that these germs were "opportunistic" infections that developed *after* fat had caused the plaque to develop.

PRIMARY VERSUS OPPORTUNISTIC PATHOGENS

Germs can be described roughly as either "primary" pathogens, germs that can attack anyone, or "opportunistic" pathogens that only attack people who are injured or weak. Primary pathogens such as HIV get the lion's share of attention, and most of the money spent on germ research is spent on them. Opportunistic infections get much less attention.

The distinction between these two kinds of germs is extremely important for people with heart disease. If your doctor believes that CPN is an opportunistic infection that only infects the arteries of people who already have heart disease, then he or she is not going to be very interested in eradicating CPN infections.

To find out whether CPN is a primary, direct cause of atherosclerosis or just an opportunistic germ that shows up later, Dr. Shor and a colleague, Dr. James Phillips, examined three types of atheromas:

- Fatty streaks (This is the earliest visible form of atheroma, and it is often found during autopsies of teenagers and young soldiers.)
- Mature atherosclerotic plaques
- Advanced plaques

Here are some of their findings:[4]

- Atherosclerosis begins when CPN destroys smooth muscle cells in arteries.
- CPN is found in early, mature, and advanced atherosclerosis.
- CPN destroys the fibers that enable muscles to contract.
- CPN makes smooth muscle cells rupture and disintegrate.
- Large numbers of CPN organisms are found in the debris created by the rupture of smooth muscle cells.
- Fatty streaks are formed by macrophages that are drawn to debris from ruptured smooth muscle cells.
- Macrophages eat the debris and CPN organisms that spill out of ruptured smooth muscle cells. (This is one of the ways that macrophages become infected with CPN.)

This study added a lot of weight to the arguments that CPN organisms are primary pathogens and that they are a direct cause of atheroslerosis.

About now, a careful reader ought to be thinking: "If CPN destroys our smooth muscle cells, it seems like our arteries would relax or rupture, our blood pressure would drop, and we would die in weeks instead of decades." Another way of stating this is: "Why doesn't CPN kill us as quickly as the Ebola virus does?"

The reason that CPN doesn't kill us in a few weeks is that CPN and humans have an exquisitely balanced relationship with each other that has evolved over many centuries, and at the expense of countless human lives. At the same time that CPN is killing some smooth muscle cells, it is releasing chemicals that make other smooth muscle cells reproduce and grow. The result is that after CPN kills millions of these cells, there are millions more of them than there were before the infection started. These new smooth muscle cells do not just replace dead ones, they grow wildly in every direction, migrating from the middle layers of our arteries into the inner and outer layers. The result is that the walls of our arteries become chaotic, thick, stiff, sticky, weak, and riddled with millions of dead macrophages. In other words, our arteries become atherosclerotic *after* they are infected with CPN.

CRP IS A MARKER FOR CPN INFECTIONS

Clay Johnston and several of his colleagues from the University of California at San Francisco performed a small but important study. Before I can tell you what they did and what they found, we need to go over some background information.

C-reactive protein (CRP) levels indicate the amount of inflammation present in our bodies. People with obesity, diabetes, and high blood pressure have high levels of CRP, so it isn't much of a surprise to find that people with atherosclerosis also have high levels of CRP.

An *endarterectomy* is an operation in which instruments are inserted into an artery to clear out atherosclerotic plaques. When everything goes right, the loose pieces of plaque are sucked out of the artery before they can block smaller arteries.

Patients with CPN infections tend to have atherosclerosis in their carotid arteries. Since the carotid arteries are close to the surface of the neck and easy to reach, carotid endarterectomies are fairly common.

Serology (antibody) tests are often used to determine whether a person is infected with a particular germ. These tests are not very accurate, but they have some value and they are used a lot. Another way of finding out if someone is infected with germ X is to collect tissue or blood specimens from the person, place the specimens in specially prepared laboratory dishes, then wait and see if germ X grows in any of the dishes. If germ X does grow, then the tissue specimens from which it grew are said to have *viable* germ X organisms. If viable germ X organisms are found in your blood, it is a sure sign that you are infected with germ X.

Now we can get back to Dr. Johnston's study. To see if CPN infections and high CRP levels were associated with each other in people with atherosclerosis, Dr. Johnston and his colleagues measured the CRP levels and CPN antibodies of forty-eight patients who were about to have carotid endarterectomies. After the endarterectomies, the researchers placed some of the plaque scrapings in laboratory dishes to see if they could grow CPN. They found viable CPN in eighteen (38 percent) of the forty-eight plaques. When all of their data was analyzed, Dr. Johnston and his colleagues discovered that the presence of high levels of CRP predicted CPN infection better than CPN serology tests did. The researchers concluded:

> Viable C. pneumoniae are present in a substantial portion of carotid artery atherosclerotic plaques and are associated with increased serum C-reactive protein levels. These findings may explain the link between elevated C-reactive protein levels and the risk of cardiovascular disease and stroke but should be reproduced in a larger cohort.[5]

Dr. Johnston's study is important for the following reasons:

- It demonstrates that high CRP levels are linked to CPN infections, suggesting that CPN is a major source of inflammation.
- It reinforces other research linking CRP and CPN to atherosclerosis.
- It strongly reinforces other research showing that serology tests alone are not enough to determine whether or not a person has a serious CPN infection.

I want to emphasize this last item. If you ask your doctor to test you for CPN, what you will probably get is a serology test. As previously mentioned, these tests are unreliable when used to identify intracellular germs, and a false negative from one of these tests could delay a proper diagnosis for years, assuming, of course, that you live for years.

If you are tested for both CRP and CPN, you have a chance of learning something important about the state of your health. If your CRP levels are high, then you have a high level of inflammation. If your CPN antibodies are also high, then there is a good chance the inflammation comes from a CPN infection.

If your CRP levels are high and your CPN antibodies are low, then you

Remember This!

When all of their data was analyzed, Dr. Johnston and his colleagues discovered that the presence of high levels of CRP predicted CPN infection better than CPN serology tests did.

may or may not have a serious CPN infection. You might be infected with CMV or another herpes virus. You might even be infected with that rare tropical parasite I thought I had picked up in Brazil.

The reason that I distinguish between a CPN infection and a *serious* CPN infection is that most older people have antibodies against CPN in their blood, but many of them are still slender and healthy. Since you're reading this book, there is a good chance you don't feel very healthy, and thus there is a good chance that your chronic infections, whatever they are, are serious. A CRP test can tell you how serious your infections are—it just can't tell you what kind they are.

There are different kinds of tests for CRP, so I can't give you a figure for what your test results should be. CRP is barely detectable in healthy young people, and it shouldn't be much higher in healthy old people.

To summarize the role of infections in atherosclerosis, germs trigger acute phase responses (APRs), and the APRs send macrophages and other immune cells into our arteries to kill the germs. The arteries become inflamed, macrophages turn into foam cells, and a fatty plaque grows where the smooth muscles and endothelial cells used to be. Cortisol contributes to this process.

CORTISOL-LIKE MEDICINES AND ATHEROSCLEROSIS

Cortisol is in a class of hormones called *corticosteroids*, and synthetic corticosteroids have been used to treat inflammatory and autoimmune diseases since the 1940s. Cortisol-like medicines make people feel better for a while, and they sometimes save lives, but patients often pay a heavy price in future suffering for any good they get from them. The terrible side effects of these drugs are described by the U.S. National Institute of Arthritis and Musculoskeletal and Skin Diseases (NIAMS) as follows:

> [Possible side effects of corticosteroids] include changes in appearance (such as acne or increased facial hair); development of a round or moon-shaped face; thin, fragile skin that bruises easily; or movement of body fat to the trunk. You might also experience mood changes, personality changes, irritability, agitation, or depression. Other possible side effects include increased appetite and weight gain, poor wound healing, headache, glaucoma, irregular menstrual periods, peptic ulcer, muscle weakness, osteoporosis, steroid-induced diabetes, and osteonecrosis (damage to the hip joint that leads to severe arthritis).[6]

If you recall the disorders that Dr. Cushing found in Miss M.G., you will notice that natural and synthetic corticosteroids cause many of the same disorders.

One of the diseases treated by synthetic corticosteroids is systemic lupus erythematosus (SLE). In the early 1970s, Drs.Bulkley and Roberts studied the effects of corticosteroids on the hearts of SLE patients. They divided the patients into two groups: patients who had been treated with corticosteroids for *less* than one year and patients who had been treated with corticosteroids for *more* than one year. These two groups were compared with each other, and with patients who had never been treated with corticosteroids.

The researchers looked at clinical and autopsy data for all three groups, and here are some of their findings:[7]

- Patients treated with corticosteroids were eight times more likely than untreated patients to experience congestive heart failure.
- Sixty-four percent of the corticosteroid-treated patients developed left ventricular hypertrophy (dangerous swellings of their hearts).
- Forty-two percent of the patients treated with corticosteroids for more than a year had partially blocked coronary arteries, and four of these patients had heart attacks. None of the patients who were treated for less than a year had blocked coronary arteries.
- Patients treated with corticosteroids were five times as likely as untreated patients to have high blood pressure.
- Patients treated with corticosteroids for more than a year were twice as likely to have high blood pressure as patients treated for less than a year.

The corticosteroids had some positive effects, of course, or they would not have been used, but the results of their study led Drs. Bulkley and Roberts to conclude: "Although vital to the management of SLE, corticosteroids have an over-all deleterious effect on the heart."[8]

NATURALLY OCCURRING CORTISOL AND ATHEROSCLEROSIS

Cortisol-like medicines unequivocally cause or exacerbate heart disease. Can naturally produced cortisol do the same? Yes. Most people with untreated Cushing's syndrome will die of heart disease, and any excess cortisol increases the risk of heart disease. In 1977, Raymond Troxler and his colleagues published a paper showing a clear link between cortisol and atherosclerosis in U.S. Air Force personnel. Here is the abstract of their paper:

> To study the association of plasma cortisol and coronary atherosclerosis, we elected 71 male outpatients who had coronary angiography as part of their evaluation at our facility. Forty-eight percent of the angiograms showed no evidence of coronary artery disease (CAD), 20% showed mild CAD, and 32% showed moderate to severe CAD. We found significant correlations between elevated serial morning plasma cortisols and moderate to severe coronary atherosclerosis. Using the odds ratio, we compared plasma cortisol to the major risk factors for coronary artery disease. Plasma cortisol was second only to serum cholesterol as a discriminator in our patient population between diseased and non-diseased patients. We found a significant correlation between plasma cortisol and cholesterol, blood pressure, and smoking—the three cardinal risk factors for CAD. The highest degree of correlation was found between cortisol and cholesterol. . . . [9]

Dr. Troxler and his colleagues found a strong link between cortisol and cholesterol, and other researchers have found the same thing.[10] Cortisol raises cholesterol levels.

CORTISOL, OBESITY, AND ATHEROSCLEROSIS

There is no doubt that cortisol-like medicines caused several kinds of heart disease in the SLE patients described by Drs. Bulkley and Roberts. When I first read the paper by Dr. Troxler and his colleagues, I assumed that excess cortisol caused the atherosclerosis they found in their Air Force patients.

When I learned that atherosclerosis begins in childhood, long before most of us show any signs of hypercortisolism, I began to wonder if atherosclerosis could raise cortisol levels. The answer seems to be yes. In a 1999 article, John Yudkin and his colleagues described how inflammatory cytokines are produced by atherosclerotic arteries. Near the end of their abstract, they state:

> Circulating IL-6 stimulates the hypothalamic-pituitary-adrenal (HPA) axis, activation of which is associated with central obesity, hypertension and insulin resistance.[11]

The *HPA axis* regulates cortisol production. In plain English, perhaps plainer than Dr. Yudkin would use, these researchers are saying that atherosclerosis stimulates cortisol production, which then leads to obesity, high blood pressure, and insulin resistance.

After reading thousands of abstracts and papers on cortisol, obesity, and atherosclerosis, I can summarize the relationship between heart disease and obesity in a single sentence: *Heart disease causes obesity as much as obesity causes heart disease.*

SUMMARY

Atherosclerosis appears to be another disease that, after being initiated by germs, develops its own self-sustaining downhill clinical course.[12] In other words, we have a vicious cycle in which hypercortisolism and atherosclerosis cause each other. Here is the way it works:

1. Cortisol reduces the ability of macrophages to kill germs, and some macrophages become infected by germs they are unable kill.
2. The infected macrophages cannot process cholesterol properly, so they turn into foam cells, swell up, and die.
3. The dead foam cells are still infected with living germs, so any healthy macrophage that tries to remove a dead one becomes infected, turns into a foam cell, and dies.
4. Dead foam cells accumulate in large clusters that we call pus and doctors call atherosclerotic lesions.
5. Dead foam cells are highly inflammatory, so healthy cells near the dead ones send out IL-6 and other cytokines that increase cortisol production.
6. The extra cortisol:
   a) Weakens the ability of macrophages to kill germs and process cholesterol.
   b) Increases the amount of cholesterol available for macrophages to choke on.
   c) Makes fat accumulate around our waists (Chapters 8–11).
7. Return to step 1.

These events repeat themselves, decade after decade, until an important artery is blocked and the cycle is stopped by death. Diet, exercise, and cholesterol-lowering drugs may reduce the speed at which this cycle repeats itself, but they cannot kill the germs that start the cycle and keep it running. Atherosclerosis will be eliminated when the germs that cause it are eradicated.

RECOMMENDED READING

The Heart Attack Germ: Prevent Strokes, Heart Attacks and the Symptoms of Alzheimer's by Protecting Yourself from the Infections and Inflammation of Cardiovascular Disease, by Louis A. Dvonch, M.D., and Russell Dvonch (Writer's Showcase, 2003).

This clearly written and well illustrated book provides useful information about C. pneumoniae *and heart disease.*

Solved: The Riddle of Heart Attacks, by Broda and Charlotte Barnes (Fries Communications, 1976).

This fine little book blames thyroid deficiencies for many of the health problems that are now attributed to excess cortisol. The authors were careful to note, however, that cortisol suppresses thyroid production. This book also presents a novel explanation for the great increase in heart disease seen in the twentieth century.

REFERENCES

Epigraph: Liuba P, Persson J, Luoma J, et al. Acute infections in children are accompanied by oxidative modification of LDL and decrease of HDL cholesterol, and are followed by thickening of carotid intima–media. *European Heart Journal* 2003; 24: 515–521.

1. *The American Heritage Dictionary of the English Language,* 4th ed. Houghton Mifflin Company, 2000.

2. Shor, Allan. Personal communication, May 17, 1999.

3. Byrne GI and Kalayoglu MV. *Chlamydia pneumoniae* and atherosclerosis: Links to the disease process. *Am Heart J* 1999 Nov;138(5 Pt 2):488–490.

4. Shor A and Phillips JI. Histological and ultrastructural findings suggesting an initiating role for *Chlamydia pneumoniae* in the pathogenesis of atherosclerosis. *Cardiovasc J S Afr* 2000 Feb;11(1):16–23.

5. Johnston SC, Messina LM, Browner WS, et al. C-reactive protein levels and viable *Chlamydia pneumoniae* in carotid artery atherosclerosis. *Stroke* 2001 Dec 1;32(12):2748–2752.

6. Patient Information Sheet #14, LUPUS: A Patient Care Guide for Nurses and Other Health Professionals. National Institute of Arthritis and Musculoskeletal and Skin Diseases, January 26, 1999.

7. Bulkley BH and Roberts WC. The heart in systemic lupus erythematosus and the changes induced in it by corticosteroid therapy. A study of 36 necropsy patients. *Am J Med* 1975 Feb;58(2):243–264.

8. Ibid. p. 243.

9. Troxler RG, Sprague EA, Albanese RA, et al. The association of elevated plasma cortisol and early atherosclerosis as demonstrated by coronary angiography. *Atherosclerosis* 1977 Feb;26(2):151–162 . *Abstract reprinted with permission of Elsevier, Ltd.*

10. Nanjee MN and Miller NE. Plasma lipoproteins and adrenocortical hormones in men—positive association of low density lipoprotein cholesterol with plasma cortisol concentration. *Clin Chim Acta* 1989 Feb 28;180(2):113–120.

11. Yudkin JS, Kumari M, Humphries SE, et al. Inflammation, obesity, stress and coronary heart disease: Is interleukin-6 the link? *Atherosclerosis* 1999 Feb;148(2): 209–214.

12. Da Prato RA and Rothschild J. The AIDS virus as an opportunistic organism inducing a state of chronic relative cortisol excess: Therapeutic implications. *Med Hypotheses* 1986 Nov;21(3):253–266.

5 Cholesterol Is Good for You

The diet-heart hypothesis has been repeatedly shown to be wrong, and yet, for complicated reasons of pride, profit and prejudice, the hypothesis continues to be exploited by scientists, fund-raising enterprises, food companies and even governmental agencies. The public is being deceived by the greatest health scam of the century.

—GEORGE V. MANN
CORONARY HEART DISEASE: THE DIETARY SENSE AND NONSENSE

The *diet-heart hypothesis* says that we can reduce our chances of having a stroke or a heart attack by reducing our consumption of cholesterol and saturated fats. Is this hypothesis true, or is it, as Dr. Mann says, the greatest health scam of the twentieth century?

It is true that people with high levels of cholesterol are slightly more likely to have strokes and heart attacks.[1] But in the previous chapter we saw that atherosclerosis, the main cause of strokes and heart attacks, begins in childhood, many years before we have high cholesterol. We also saw that atherosclerosis is caused by infections and cortisol, and we saw that cortisol and cholesterol levels are closely linked to each other. It appears that infections cause both atherosclerosis and high cholesterol levels.

Atheromas, the sores that form in our arteries, contain large amounts of cholesterol, but most of that cholesterol is carried into the atheromas by foam cells. The most important foam cells are macrophages that have been crippled by infections and excess cortisol. Foam cells are probably *not* created by high cholesterol levels.[2,3]

The diet-heart hypothesis has convinced many people that cholesterol is dangerous, but it is actually good for us. Cholesterol reinforces our cell membranes, protects our nerve cells, and helps us to digest our food. All of our steroid hormones, including cortisol and our sex hormones, are made from it. When our cholesterol levels are low we are more likely to suffer from infections, cancer, anemia, hyperthyroidism, or liver disease, or to experience an early death.[4]

The question of cholesterol is an important one, and eventually each of us will have to decide whether to reduce, raise, or ignore our cholesterol levels. The issue is too complicated to be settled here, but I want to give you some information in this chapter you are not likely to see anywhere else.

THE PROS AND CONS OF LOWERING CHOLESTEROL

In Chapter 4, I explained how dying macrophages turn into foam cells and carry cholesterol into our blood vessels. If nothing else kills us first, the dead macrophages will eventually block a major artery. The standard method of slowing this process is to reduce the amount of cholesterol in the blood to such a low level that only a few macrophages can turn into foam cells. When we consider the many benefits we get from cholesterol, we have to ask ourselves: "Is cholesterol reduction the best way to keep our arteries open?"

To help us explore this question, let's try a brief thought experiment. Thought experiments don't prove anything, but they often give us new perspectives on old problems. In this case, imagine that you are a lawmaker in a frontier state where the ranchers often lynch suspected horse thieves.

You and your fellow legislators, after much deep thought and many committee meetings, decide that the best way to end your lynching problem is to reduce the availability of rope. You start an education campaign to discourage people from using rope. You put warning labels on ropes, and you require every rope to be registered. Your sheriffs make sudden midnight raids on suspected rope dealers. After a while, ropes become so hard to find that rope-mediated mortality (hanging) drops a little. Not much, but enough to be statistically significant.

Unfortunately, your new law has some unwanted side effects. Dirty, long-haired rope dealers sneak around schoolyards trying to sell rope to your children. Sheriffs have frequent shootouts with rope dealers. Ranchers soon learn that they can hang a horse thief with a chain as easily as they can with a rope. Soon your legislative analysts report that *overall* mortality—the total number of people dying in your state—is up sharply even though there are fewer hangings. Furthermore, the cost of your war against rope has bankrupted your state. You close some schools and begin another round of deep thinking.

Does this war against rope sound silly? Well, it is no sillier than our war against cholesterol. Cholesterol has the same relationship to heart disease that a rope has to a lynching—it is part of the process, but it is by no means the cause of the process. Reducing cholesterol prevents a few deaths from heart attacks, but it increases the number of deaths from other causes.

In a group of people who are at high risk for heart attacks, lowering cholesterol will save a few more than it kills. In a group at low risk, lowering cholesterol will kill a few more than it saves. In either case, there is little difference in the *number* killed, but there is a big difference in *who* is killed. Asking millions of people to lower their cholesterol levels is like asking them to play Russian roulette.

The ideal way to keep your arteries open would be to eliminate your infections and reduce your cortisol levels, but both of those things are difficult to do right now. While waiting for the ideal treatment to be developed, you and your doctor may decide that the benefits of low cholesterol outweigh the risks. Are you going to use diet or drugs? Most people begin with diet.

WHY DIETING WILL NOT LOWER YOUR CHOLESTEROL (MUCH)

Can you lower your cholesterol by eating right? No. You can only lower your cholesterol by eating wrong.

The body produces cholesterol from saturated fats, and production is regulated very carefully. If you eat a little cholesterol, your body makes a little less and your cholesterol level stays the same. If you eat a lot of it, your body makes a lot less. As far back as 1956, an expert on fat, Ancel Keys, wrote: ". . . . serum cholesterol is essentially independent of the cholesterol intake over the whole range of human diets."[5] Forty-one years later, Dr. Keys went even further:

> There's no connection whatsoever between cholesterol in food and cholesterol in blood. And we've known that all along. Cholesterol in the diet doesn't matter at all unless you happen to be a chicken or a rabbit.[6]

Cholesterol is so closely regulated that attempts to disregulate it may have paradoxical effects. William Castelli, who directed the famous Framingham study for many years, wrote:

> In Framingham, Massachusetts, the more saturated fat one ate, the more

> cholesterol one ate, the more calories one ate, the lower people's serum cholesterol. . . . we found that the people who ate the most cholesterol, ate the most saturated fat, ate the most calories, weighed the least and were the most physically active.[7]

There is a huge body of research showing that dietary fat and cholesterol are not the culprits in heart disease. Here are some comments on that research from two British experts:

> The commonly-held belief that the best diet for the prevention of coronary heart disease is a low saturated fat, low cholesterol is not supported by the available evidence from clinical trials. In the primary prevention, such diets do not reduce the risk of myocardial infarction or coronary or all cause mortality. . . .
>
> Similarly, diets focused exclusively on reduction of saturated fats and cholesterol are relatively ineffective for secondary prevention and should be abandoned. There may be other effective diets for secondary prevention of coronary heart disease but these are not yet sufficiently well defined or adequately tested. . . .[8]

"Primary prevention" is preventing first heart attacks; "secondary prevention" is preventing subsequent heart attacks.

The experts quoted so far were writing about diets that ordinary people are likely to eat. If you lock people up and make them eat whatever you give them, then you can indeed lower their cholesterol levels. The U.S. Department of Health and Human Services (DHHS) tells us how to do it:

> Demonstrating a clinical benefit of modern cholesterol-lowering diets in asymptomatic persons has proven difficult. In three controlled trials in institutionalized patients, fat-modified diets reduced serum cholesterol 12–14% with generally favorable effects on CHD [coronary heart disease] over periods of up to eight years. Each of these studies used diets high in polyunsaturated fat, which have been associated with adverse effects, and none excluded patients with CHD. As a result, their findings may not be applicable to currently recommended low-fat diets in asymptomatic persons.[9]

You are not likely to lower your cholesterol very much by dieting, so sooner or later your doctor may prescribe a cholesterol-lowering drug. The most important of these drugs are the statins.

STATINS

Unlike diets, statins reliably lower cholesterol and reduce the risk of having a heart attack. There are other ways of dying besides heart attacks, however, and if you check the advertisements for statins, you will often see a message that reads something like "This product has not been shown to increase life expectancy."

There is a small mystery associated with statins because they reduce the risk of angina and heart attack more than we would expect from lowering cholesterol levels. This paradox led researchers to discover that statins reduce the level of C-reactive protein (CRP) in the blood. This suggests that statins reduce inflammation.

If statins reduce inflammation, German researchers may have learned how they do it. In a laboratory experiment, they found that one of them, cerivastatin, reduced the rate at which *Chlamydophila pneumoniae* germs infected endothelial cells and macrophages.[10] Unfortunately, cerivastatin was taken off the market because of its side effects.[11] More research is needed to learn whether or not other statins inhibit the growth of *Chlamydophila pneumoniae.*

Caution

Statins are safer and more effective than earlier drugs, but they still have dangerous side effects and drug interactions. In Chapter 1, I described the miraculous response I had to my first course of clarithromycin. Unfortunately, clarithromycin is a "macrolide" antibiotic, and statins and macrolides should not be used together. If you are taking statins, be sure to speak to your pharmacist about possible drug interactions with any medications you may be taking or considering.

SUMMARY

Lowering cholesterol is good for some people and bad for others, and it is not easy to know which group we fall into. We need to take our doctor's advice, but we should make sure she is aware of the arguments *against* lowering cholesterol as well as the arguments *for* lowering it.

Dr. Mann, whom I quoted at the beginning of the chapter, called the diet-heart hypothesis a scam. I don't believe the hypothesis is a trick or a swindle;

it is just a tragic mistake that occurred because of historical accidents. You can read about these accidents in the books and reports listed below.

RECOMMENDED READING AND RESOURCES

The cholesterol/fat question is very complicated, and the NIH has given us oversimplified answers. The books and articles listed below give a better perspective.

The Cholesterol Myths: Exposing the Fallacy That Saturated Fat and Cholesterol Cause Heart Disease, by Uffe Ravnskov, M.D., Ph.D. (New Trends Publishing, 2000).
This small book discusses many popular misconceptions about cholesterol. Purchase a paper copy or download it from www.ravnskov.nu/cholesterol.htm.

Heart Failure: A Critical Inquiry into American Medicine and the Revolution in Heart Care, by Thomas J. Moore (Random House, 1989).
This book reveals the dismal results of research on heart disease since World War II. All of Mr. Moore's health books are interesting and valuable.

"The Low Fat/Low Cholesterol Diet is Ineffective," by Laura Corr and Michael Oliver (*European Heart Journal* 1997;18:18–22).
This fascinating report is available at www.omen.com/corr.html and it is well worth the few minutes it takes to read.

Oils in Context, by Raymond Peat.
This report presents some eye-opening facts about fats. Available from www.efn.org/~raypeat/oils.rtf.

"The Epidemic That Wasn't?"; "What If Americans Ate Less Saturated Fat?"; and "The Soft Science of Dietary Fat," by Gary Taubes (*Science,* March 30, 2001).
If you still think that fat causes heart disease, read these articles by Gary Taubes in the March 30, 2001, issue of Science.

REFERENCES

Epigraph: Mann, George V. *Coronary Heart Disease: The Dietary Sense and Nonsense.* London: Veritas Society, 1993.

1. National Institutes of Health. 2002 Sept. Final Report National Cholesterol Education Program National Heart, Lung, and Blood Institute. *Third Report of the National Cholesterol Education Program (NCEP) Expert Panel on Detection, Evaluation, and Treatment of High Blood Cholesterol in Adults (Adult Treatment Panel III).* NIH Publication No. 02-5215.

2. Cheng W, Kvilekval KV, and Abumrad NA. Dexamethasone enhances accu-

mulation of cholesteryl esters by human macrophages. *Am J Physiol* 1995 Oct; 269(4 Pt 1):E642–E648.

3. Cheng W, Lau OD, and Abumrad NA. Two antiatherogenic effects of progesterone on human macrophages; inhibition of cholesteryl ester synthesis and block of its enhancement by glucocorticoids. *J Clin Endocrinol Metab* 1999 Jan;84(1): 265–271.

4. National Institutes of Health. 1994 Apr. *Physiology and Pathology of Low Cholesterol States.* NIH Guide PA-94-057, Vol 23, No. 15.

5. Keys A. The diet and the development of coronary heart disease. *J Chronic Dis.* 1956 Oct;4(4):364–380.

6. Keys A. *Eating Well.* 1997 March/April.

7. Castelli WP. Concerning the possibility of a nut . . . *Arch Intern Med* 1992 July;152(7):1371–2. Quoted in www.mercola.com/2001/aug/4/oil.htm.

8. Corr LA and Oliver MF. The low fat/low cholesterol diet is ineffective. *European Heart Journal* 1997; 18: 18–22.

9. "Screening for High Blood Cholesterol and Other Lipid Abnormalities." U.S. Department of Health and Human Sevices. http://odphp.osophs.dhhs.gov/pubs/guidecps/text/CH02.txt.

10. Kothe H, Dalhoff K, Rupp J, et al. Hydroxymethylglutaryl coenzyme A reductase inhibitors modify the inflammatory response of human macrophages and endothelial cells infected with *Chlamydia pneumoniae. Circulation* 2000 Apr 18; 101(15): 1760–1763.

11. Cerivastatin. MedLine Plus. www.nlm.nih.gov/medlineplus/druginfo/med master/a600044.html.

6

Hypertension Is Not All Bad

It has been a matter of wonder to me to see the extraordinary resourcefulness of those who treat blood-pressure and the numerous theories that guide them. The drugs that have been employed are legion in number, diets of the most contrary descriptions—all-flesh diet, vegetarian diet, purin-free diet, and various other modifications; baths and waters and exercises of all kinds; . . . Notwithstanding this the blood-pressure has remained high.

—SIR JAMES MACKENZIE, M.D.
PRINCIPLES OF DIAGNOSIS AND TREATMENT IN HEART AFFECTATIONS, 1917

Sir James's grim observations about blood pressure are as true today as they were during World War I, except that today there are even more theories, drugs, and diets. Chronically high blood pressure—*hypertension*—is still a major health problem.

The main reason that we have made so little progress in treating hypertension is because it is still treated like a disease when it is, in most cases, a life-saving response to other health problems. Hypertension helps us survive infections, stress, obesity, and atherosclerosis.

Unfortunately, the help we get from hypertension often comes at the cost of strokes, kidney failure, and heart failure.

HOW HYPERTENSION COMPENSATES FOR INFECTIONS

In January of 1999 my blood pressure was typically 160/100 mm Hg (millimeters of mercury) without medication, and not much better with medication. In April of 1999, a few weeks after completing the clarithromycin treatment described in Chapter 1, my blood pressure was down to 117/74 mm Hg without medications. The nurses at my giant HMO joked that I had the blood pressure of a teenager. I didn't know anything about inflammations or cortisol at the time, so I was completely mystified by the fact that an antibiotic had lowered my blood pressure. Now it is easy to understand.

Infections cause inflammations, and inflammations cause our blood vessels to dilate. The dilated vessels allow more blood to flow through inflamed tissues, and the extra blood contributes to faster healing. At the same time, because of our dilated blood vessels, our blood pressure drops. A serious inflammation can reduce our blood pressure to dangerously low levels.

The same inflammations that dilate our blood vessels also trigger the release of cortisol. Cortisol constricts our blood vessels and reduces the amount of blood that can flow through them. This compensates for the dilated vessels and raises our blood pressure.

Cortisol often under- or over-compensates for dilation, so any particular infection may either reduce or raise our blood pressure. Generally, serious, acute infections lower our blood pressure, but milder, long-term infections raise our blood pressure. Figure 6.1 shows how infections and inflammations contribute to hypertension.

I believe my blood pressure fell in 1999 because I was temporarily free from my long-term *Chlamydophila pneumoniae* (CPN) infection, and my cortisol level had returned to normal. When my CPN symptoms returned, both my cortisol level and my blood pressure rose again.

HOW HYPERTENSION COMPENSATES FOR STRESS

Blood carries oxygen and nutrients to our muscles and organs. In emergencies, when we might have to fight or flee, blood is diverted away from some muscles and organs to provide more blood to others. Consequently, during emergencies, our overall blood pressure must rise to ensure that all of our organs and muscles get the oxygen and nutrients they need.

People in wealthy, industrialized countries seldom face real emergencies, but we face almost constant annoyances from telephones, traffic, taxes, noise, and so on. Coping with these annoyances requires alertness and action, and our blood pressure rises to help us get through our stress-filled days. When we are healthy, our blood pressure drops in the evening.

Our blood pressure is so important, and the task of controlling it is so difficult, that we have evolved at least six systems to do it. These systems are heavily biased toward keeping our blood pressure higher rather than lower.

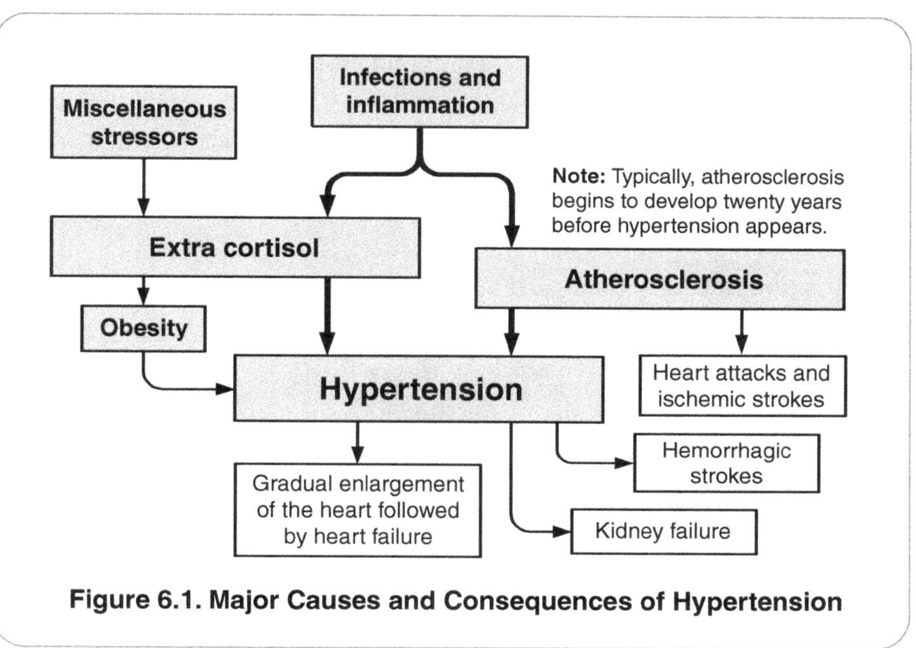

Figure 6.1. Major Causes and Consequences of Hypertension

At first, this sounds like a pretty poor design, but it meets our survival needs very well because low blood pressure is much more dangerous than high blood pressure. Low blood pressure can kill us in a few minutes, but high blood pressure allows us to lead normal, active lives for many years.

Two stress hormones, norepinephrine and cortisol, raise our blood pressure during times of stress, and a chronic excess of either hormone leads to hypertension.

HOW HYPERTENSION COMPENSATES FOR OBESITY

As we gain weight, we grow new blood vessels to supply additional blood to our fat cells. If our circulatory system was a simple hydraulic system, made up of pumps and hoses, these new hoses (blood vessels) would make our blood pressure drop.

Fortunately, our circulatory system contains a feedback loop that raises our blood pressure as we gain weight. Fat cells produce a hormone called leptin, and our leptin level increases as we accumulate fat. Leptin raises our blood pressure to compensate for the extra load that obesity places on our circulatory system. With the help of leptin and hypertension, we can live long and well even when we are seriously overweight. We might live longer and better if we were thin, but that is not an option for many of us.

HOW HYPERTENSION COMPENSATES FOR ATHEROSCLEROSIS

People with hypertension tend to have the following kinds of atherosclerotic damage to their arteries:

- Excessive numbers of smooth muscle cells (hyperplasia)
- Migration of smooth muscle cells from middle layers to inner layers of blood vessels
- Endothelial cells that cannot control the contraction and relaxation of smooth muscle cells
- Increased thickness of blood vessel walls
- Scar tissue in the middle and outer layers
- Movement of macrophages and other immune cells into the walls of arteries[1]

The disorders listed above begin to appear when we are children, long before our blood pressure starts climbing. The damage first appears in a few arteries and then slowly spreads throughout our body, and as it spreads, our arteries become stiffer and stiffer. Blood does not flow very well through stiff arteries, so the brain, which controls blood pressure, gradually increases our blood pressure to keep blood flowing through all of our organs and muscles. Because of the extra blood pressure, we feel good and stay active despite the damage to our arteries.

High blood pressure compensates for infections, stress, obesity, and hardening of the arteries, and all four of these disorders can be traced back to middle-path germs like the ones discussed in Chapters 3 and 4.

MEDICINES USED TO TREAT HYPERTENSION

When our blood pressure first starts to climb, our doctors prod us to exercise more and eat less. Exercise and diet almost never lower anyone's blood pressure, so our doctors eventually prescribe antihypertensive drugs.

The ideal antihypertensive medicine would cure our infections, lower our stress level, help us lose weight, and repair our arteries. No such drug is available yet, of course, so doctors are forced to prescribe drugs that drive our blood pressure down without regard to the problems that are raising our blood pressure. I've been treated with eight of these medicines, and none of them lowered my blood pressure very much, and they all had dangerous or unpleasant side effects. Research suggests that my experience was typical.

The medicines I took had little effect on my blood pressure for two reasons. First, they had little or no effect on my infections, stress, obesity, or atherosclerosis. Second, each medicine targeted only one of the six blood-pressure control systems. Let's do a short thought experiment and see what happens when we try to suppress the wrong system.

Imagine that you have high blood pressure and it is caused by too much cortisol. The chance that your doctor will diagnose this problem correctly is essentially zero, so she will be forced to guess which medicine will work best for you. Let's imagine further that the first medicine your doctor tries is a beta blocker. The nerve signals to your heart are weakened, your heart beats less vigorously, and your blood pressure drops a little.

Within a few days, you feel like you are pulling an anchor behind you when you walk, but this is just the beginning. The other five systems that control your blood pressure sense a drop in blood pressure, so they try to raise it back to what it was. If they succeed, your doctor will increase your dose of beta blocker until your blood pressure stays down. Now your body is flooded with chemicals that are trying to raise your blood pressure and other chemicals that are trying to lower it. You may begin to experience beta-blocker side effects. These include coughing, depression, dizziness, hallucinations, low blood sugar, impotence, insomnia, kidney function impairment, lightheadedness, liver impairment, and nightmares.[2]

After a few weeks, your doctor takes you off of the beta blocker and makes another guess. This guessing game goes on until she stumbles onto a medicine that lowers your blood pressure without making you feel too awful. Unless you insist, your cortisol levels will never be measured. If your cortisol levels are measured, there is a good chance that the wrong methods will be used or the results will be misinterpreted. Chapters 15 and 16 discuss these problems.

SUMMARY

Our bodies compensate for several kinds of health problems by raising our blood pressure, and the extra blood pressure can itself cause serious illnesses. When our blood pressure becomes very high, we will need some kind of anti-hypertensive medicine.

When taking these medicines, keep in mind that the antihypertensive medicines available in 2005 do not cure anything. They may help you live longer, but to get well you need to correct the problems that cause hypertension: infections, stress, obesity, and atherosclerosis.

RECOMMENDED RESOURCE

Hearts & Arteries (National Institute on Aging, 1994).

This is an excellent introduction to the circulatory system. Available from www.niapublications.org/pubs/ hearts-arteries/index.asp.

REFERENCES

Epigraph: Mackenzie, James. *Principles of Diagnosis and Treatment in Heart Affectations.* London, Oxford Medical Publications, 1917, p. 204.

1. National Institutes of Health. Cellular and Molecular Interrelationships of Atherosclerosis and Hypertension; NIH Guide. NHLBI RFA HL-98-009.

2. Wolfe SM, Fugate L, Hulstrand EP. *Worst Pills Best Pills.* Public Citizen Health Research Group, 1988, and other sources.

7 The Stages of Potbelly Syndrome

Perhaps the biggest problem with chronic stress and elevated cortisol levels is the fact that the initial effects are so subtle—a few extra pounds of weight, a slight reduction in energy levels, a modest drop in sex drive, a bit of trouble with memory—that we simply brush them off as "normal" aspects of aging. . . . these effects are actually the earliest signs of obesity, diabetes, impotence, dementia, heart disease, cancer, and many related conditions.

—SHAWN TALBOTT, *THE CORTISOL CONNECTION*

Potbelly syndrome (PBS) creeps up on us slowly, like old age. The symptoms have no obvious connection with each other, so we are likely to accept each new one as just another sign that we are getting older.

We almost never write down the date when we first notice a new health problem, but if we did we would find that the signs and symptoms of PBS appear in stages that correspond roughly to four well-documented medical conditions. The stages, listed from least to most serious, are: 1) Reaven's syndrome X (RSX); 2) Subclinical Cushing's syndrome (SCCS); 3) Dysmetabolic syndrome X (DSX); 4) Type 2 diabetes.

This division into four stages, instead of three or six or ten, is the result of historical accidents, not a well-thought-out plan. The names are also accidents of time and place; that's why some of them sound a little odd.

Table 7.1 lists the major disorders linked to each stage. Since PBS and Cushing's syndrome (CS) are both caused by excess cortisol, the symptoms of CS are listed for comparison. In real people, progression from one stage to the next is not as orderly as it appears in the table. Sleep disorders, for example, are common in all stages of PBS. Still, the table provides a fairly good picture of how PBS develops.

TABLE 7.1. DISORDERS ASSOCIATED WITH POTBELLY SYNDROME

	Potbelly Syndrome Stages					
Disorders	**RSX**	**SCCS**	**DSX**	**Diabetes**	**CS**	**You?**
DISORDERS LINKED TO SMALL EXCESSES OF CORTISOL						
Insulin resistance	■	■	■	■	■	
High blood pressure	■	■	■	■	■	
High insulin levels	■	■	■	■	■	
Blood-fat (lipid) problems	■	■	■	■	■	
Cholesterol problems	■	■	■	■	■	
Blood-clotting problems	■		■	■	■	
Obesity, diffuse		■	■	■		
High glucose levels		■	■	■	■	
Eye problems		■	■	■	■	
Excessive hunger/thirst		■		■	■	
Frequent urination		■		■	■	
DISORDERS LINKED TO MODERATE OR LONG-TERM EXCESSES OF CORTISOL						
Many infections & coinfections			■	■	■	
Obesity, abdominal			■	■	■	
Depression/fatigue/lethargy			■	■	■	
Kidney failure			■	■	■	
Heart disease			■	■	■	
Heart attacks			■	■	■	
Strokes			■	■	■	
Extremely high glucose levels				■		
Glucose in urine				■		
DISORDERS LINKED TO SEVERE OR VERY LONG-TERM EXCESSES OF CORTISOL						
Sleep disorders					■	
Major psychiatric problems					■	
Moon face					■	
Fat on back ("buffalo" hump)					■	
Skin bruises easily					■	
Muscles are weak and thin					■	
Bones break easily					■	

Legend: CS = Cushing's syndrome; Diabetes = type 2 diabetes; DSX = dysmetabolic syndrome X; RSX = Reaven's syndrome X; SCCS = subclinical Cushing's syndrome

With a few changes, Table 7.1 could be called "Disorders Associated with Insulin Resistance" because insulin resistance is the mechanism by which cortisol causes most of the symptoms of potbelly syndrome. The next chapter will explain how a small excess of cortisol can trigger the cascade of disorders listed in Table 7.1.

STAGE 1. REAVEN'S SYNDROME X (RSX)

RSX is potbelly syndrome before the potbelly appears. People with RSX, and nothing worse, look great and feel fine because their current health problems cannot be seen or felt. Their future health problems can be predicted by laboratory tests, but these tests are almost never performed on people who look good and feel well.

STAGE 2. SUBCLINICAL CUSHING'S SYNDROME (SCCS)

By the time people develop SCCS, they are beginning to look and feel unwell. This is when they start to read diet books. They jog, take vitamins, and get regular checkups. Doctors treat their symptoms with the latest wonder drugs. Still, every year they gain weight and feel a little worse than they did the year before.

SCCS was first described as an illness caused by small adrenal tumors called *incidentalomas*. These tumors are usually found by accident in patients who are examined by ultrasound or computed tomography (CT) for other reasons. Patients with incidentalomas are often classified as having *subtle hypercortisolism* because their blood cortisol levels seldom exceed the NIH's reference range of 5 to 25 µg/dL (micrograms per deciliter). Many infections raise cortisol levels above those found in patients with incidentalomas, so it is reasonable to include stress- or infection-induced SCCS as an early stage of the potbelly syndrome.

Rossi and colleagues examined fifty patients with incidentalomas. As shown in Table 7.2, many of them had serious health problems. The subset of twelve patients who met their strict definition of SCCS were in even worse condition.[1]

All of the patients who were treated for their hypercortisolism improved. Without the happy accidents that revealed their incidentalomas, there is virtually no chance that these patients would have ever been diagnosed correctly.

How many people have incidentalomas? No one knows for sure, but Marchesa and colleagues found that 7.4 percent of the patients undergoing

TABLE 7.2. HEALTH PROBLEMS OF PEOPLE WITH SUBTLE HYPERCORTISOLISM

Health Problems	All Fifty Patients	Twelve Patients with SCCS
Mild to severe hypertension	48%	92%
Obesity	36%	50%
Abnormal lipids (fats)	28%	50%
Type 2 diabetes	24%	42%
Cortisol levels	18.9 μg/dL	18.1 μg/dL

abdominal CT scans at their facility had at least one.[2] If that percentage holds true everywhere, then we would expect about 20 million Americans to have incidentalomas. We would also expect many of those people to have PBS.

STAGE 3. DYSMETABOLIC SYNDROME X (DSX)

As we get older, we accumulate more chronic infections, and the problems caused by infections and inflammation are intermingled with the problems caused by PBS. By the time people reach the DSX stage of PBS they are often obese and depressed, and many of them die from heart attacks, infections, and strokes.

This stage is sometimes called *metabolic syndrome X,* and it is one of the largest health problems in the United States. In 1999, the *Annals of the New York Academy of Science* devoted an issue to metabolic syndrome X that included an article by Barbara Hansen from the Obesity and Diabetes Research Center at the University of Maryland. Dr. Hansen wrote:

> The new millennium is likely to establish the Metabolic Syndrome X as one of the most prevalent diseases of mankind, and one of the most costly in its contributions to morbidity and premature mortality. . . . particularly from atherosclerosis and other cardiovascular diseases.[3]

Dr. Hansen discussed the prevalence of metabolic syndrome in the United States:

> In the United States, an estimate of the Metabolic Syndrome X prevalence might start with the assumption that most persons with Type 2 diabetes (in the U. S. about 12 million) are members of the Metabolic Syndrome group. One could add to this all who have a combination of obesity and impaired

> glucose tolerance (another 12 million or so in the U.S.). Those with hypertension together with some of the syndrome features might add another 10 million. It would therefore not be surprising, after deleting duplicate individuals (individuals entering into the syndrome through more than one of the above groups) that in the U.S. alone, by the year 2010, there may be among the adult population some 50 to 75 million or more with significant manifestation of this syndrome.[4]

Dr. Hansen's article is excellent. If you have several of the disorders listed in Table 7.1, it is worth a trip to your local medical library to see what she and her colleagues have to say about DSX.

STAGE 4. TYPE 2 DIABETES

Type 2 Diabetes and DSX are almost identical, except that people with diabetes have higher levels of sugar (glucose) in their blood, and they may have sugar in their urine. Both conditions are caused by excess cortisol and *mediated* by insulin resistance, that is, cortisol is the original cause of both disor-

What's in a Name?

The word *dysmetabolism* means simply "bad metabolism," and Reaven's syndrome X is therefore a *dysmetabolic syndrome.* Soon after Dr. Reaven introduced his now-famous syndrome, it became clear that there was a need for an expanded version of it to include obesity and other factors that he had intentionally omitted. Dozens of researchers have introduced their own expanded dysmetabolic syndromes, and they have used many different names.

When we defined the stages of the potbelly syndrome, we called stage three the *dysmetabolic syndrome X* (DSX), because that is the name used by the U.S. Centers for Disease Control (CDC). When we are talking about generic "bad metabolic" syndromes, we will use the term *dysmetabolic syndromes.* When we quote people directly, we will use whatever term they use.

To a great extent, the various "X" and "dysmetabolic" syndromes are just descriptions of advanced insulin resistance, so the term "insulin resistance syndrome" is slowly replacing the earlier terms.

ders, and insulin resistance is an intermediate cause. Insulin resistance and DSX will be discussed in the next chapter, and diabetes will be discussed in Chapter 13.

CUSHING'S SYNDROME (CS)

The signs and symptoms of CS are similar to those of PBS, except that CS develops more rapidly, and it is often much more severe. Most cases of CS are caused by cortisol-like medicines, not cortisol. In those cases where CS is caused by excess cortisol, the excess is usually caused by tumors, not by infections or stress. CS is discussed in Chapter 14.

HOW MANY PEOPLE HAVE POTBELLY SYNDROME?

The Centers for Disease Control in Atlanta doesn't keep track of PBS cases, yet, so we have to guess how many people have it today. Dr. Hansen estimated that by 2010 there would be 50 to 75 million people in the United States with stage 3 ([dys]metabolic syndrome X) or stage 4 (type 2 diabetes). That seems like a reasonable estimate.

Most people with hypercortisolism will have insulin resistance, and most people with insulin resistance can be assumed to have PBS. There are tens of millions of people with cortisol-stimulating infections. To them, we can add 20 million more with incidentalomas and small pituitary tumors. And then there are hundreds of thousands more who have Cushing's syndrome caused by cortisol-like medicines. I would guess that by 2010 a hundred million Americans will have PBS, with, as Dr. Hansen estimated, 50 to 75 million of them in stages 3 and 4.

If nothing changes, most of these people will be treated for obesity, high cholesterol, and hypertension until they die from heart disease, diabetes, or infection. Few of them will ever have their cortisol levels tested.

SUMMARY

The signs and symptoms of PBS develop slowly, but they appear in a predictable, consistent way, and the stages are well defined in the medical literature. The small increase in cortisol required to cause PBS is almost never detected, in part because no one ever looks for it. Insulin resistance, the intermediate cause of PBS, is almost never detected until after the patient has developed obesity, hypertension, or type 2 diabetes.

There appear to be tens of millions of Americans walking around in various stages of PBS. If that seems like a lot, stop and think about how many people you know who have potbellies.

REFERENCES

Epigraph: Tablott SM. *The Cortisol Connection: Why Stress Makes You Fat and Ruins Your Health—And What You Can Do About It*. Hunter House, 2002, pp xiii–xiv.

1. Rossi R, Tauchmanova L, Luciano A, et al. Subclinical Cushing's syndrome in patients with adrenal incidentaloma: Clinical and biochemical features. *J Clin Endocrinol Metab* 2000 Apr;85(4):1440–1448.

2. Marchesa P, Fazio VW, Church JM, et al. Adrenal masses in patients with familial adenomatous polyposis. *Dis Colon Rectum* 1997 Sep;40(9):1023–1028.

3. Hansen BC. The Metabolic Syndrome X. *Annals of the New York Academy of Sciences*. 1999 Nov 18; 892: 12–13.

This is the best summary of Syndrome X available.

4. Ibid. p. 13.

8

Infections and Insulin Resistance

. . . people who are obese are always insulin resistant.

—JACK CHALLEM ET AL., *SYNDROME X*

After a meal, our digestive system converts fats to fatty acids, proteins to amino acids, and carbohydrates to *glucose* (blood sugar). These nutrients pass into the bloodstream and eventually find their way to the places where they are needed. The most important of these substances, for our minute-to-minute survival, is glucose. The metabolic system's first priority is glucose metabolism—everything else is subordinate to the burning, storing, and retrieval of glucose.

Insulin is a hormone that lowers glucose levels by transporting glucose out of the bloodstream and into certain cells. Insulin also helps our cells burn and store glucose. *Insulin resistance* is a stress response that raises our glucose levels by interfering with the transport of glucose from blood to cells. This phenomenon was discovered about 150 years ago, and the names that have been attached to it since then reflect our growing knowledge of its effects and cause:

- *Glucosuria* of surgery (glucose found in the urine of surgical patients)
- *Hyperglycemia* of surgery (high glucose levels in the blood of surgical patients)
- Diabetes of injury (diabetes-like condition caused by trauma or infection)
- Stress diabetes (diabetes-like condition caused by stress)
- Insulin insensitivity (inability of the body to respond to insulin)
- Insulin resistance (inability of liver and muscle cells to respond to insulin)

Insulin resistance is an important part of a sequence of events that begins with chronic infections and progresses, over a period of years, to potbelly syndrome. Before we discuss insulin resistance any further, we need to review the main features of normal glucose regulation.

NORMAL, UNSTRESSED GLUCOSE REGULATION

Our glucose level begins to rise about ten minutes after we eat, and it continues to rise for another hour or two. Then it falls slowly until we eat again. This process is controlled by many hormones, but the ones of interest in this chapter are:

- Insulin, which tends to lower glucose levels.
- Glucagon, which tries to prevent glucose levels from falling too much.
- Cortisol, which raises glucose levels when we are stressed.

Glucose and hormone levels are controlled by several delicately balanced feedback loops. The loops interact with each other in various ways, and their interactions are summarized in Figures 8.1 and 8.2. Insulin resistance unbalances these feedback loops to raise glucose levels.

WHY WE BECOME INSULIN RESISTANT

At some point in our evolutionary history we developed two kinds of cells, and we developed a mechanism whereby some of those cells could be sacrificed to preserve the others. The two kinds of cells are classified as *insulin dependent* and *insulin independent*, and insulin resistance is the mechanism that sacrifices insulin-dependent cells for the benefit of insulin-independent cells.

Insulin-Dependent Cells

Insulin-dependent cells need insulin to help them "take up" glucose, fatty acids, and amino acids from the blood. When insulin and glucose are both present, insulin-dependent cells take up large amounts of glucose to burn and to store for future use. Because of their ability to store energy, these cells can survive for long periods without taking any glucose from the blood. They can also release some of their stored energy for use by other cells. Insulin-dependent cells include fat cells, liver cells, and muscle cells.

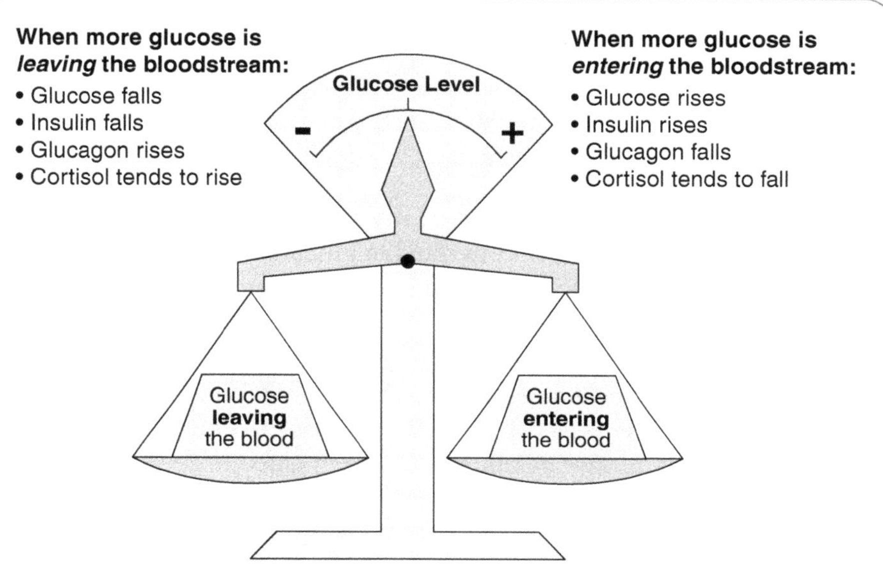

Figure 8.1. Glucose Levels Control Hormone Levels
Insulin and glucagon levels rise and fall with small changes in glucose. Cortisol levels, on the other hand, generally are not affected by small changes in glucose.

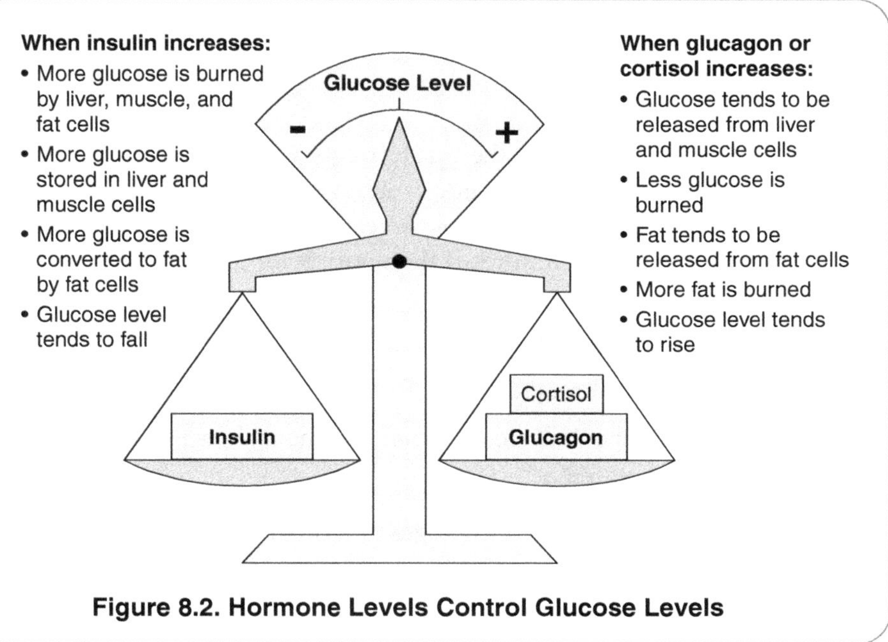

Figure 8.2. Hormone Levels Control Glucose Levels

Fat cells (adipocytes). When insulin and fatty acids are present in the blood, fat cells take up the fatty acids and convert them to fats called *triglycerides* for long-term storage. When insulin and glucose are present, fat cells convert glucose to triglycerides. When insulin and glucose levels are low, fat cells convert triglycerides back to fatty acids and release them into the bloodstream for use by other cells.

Triglycerides are made up of three fatty-acid molecules and one *glycerol* molecule. Fatty acids cannot be converted to glucose, but glycerol molecules can be metabolized by the liver to provide small amounts of glucose.

Liver cells (hepatocytes). When insulin and glucose are present, liver cells take up glucose and store it as a starch called *glycogen*. When insulin and glucose levels are low, liver cells convert glycogen back to glucose and release it into the bloodstream for use by other cells. When glucose levels are low, liver cells can break down amino acids to produce small quantities of glucose.

Muscle cells. Muscle cells behave somewhat like liver cells, except that they cannot store very much glycogen. They can, however, convert large quantities of amino acids to proteins when both insulin and amino acids are present. When glucose and fat are both scarce, muscle cells begin to convert their proteins back to amino acids. The amino acids are further metabolized to provide small amounts of glucose.

Insulin-Independent Cells

Insulin-independent cells can take up nutrients without help from insulin, but they cannot store energy, and they cannot burn fat efficiently. They begin to malfunction instantly when glucose levels fall too far, and some of them can be injured or killed in minutes if their supply of glucose is interrupted. Insulin-independent cells include:

- Brain and other nerve cells
- Red blood cells (erythrocytes)
- Endothelial cells (the delicate cells that line the insides of blood vessels)
- Eye cells (lens and retina)
- Immune cells, including macrophages and other germ-killing cells
- Kidney cells (glomeruli)
- Wound-repair cells

All of our cells are important, of course, but some of the insulin-independent cells listed above are particularly important for minute-to-minute survival. Thus it makes sense that we would evolve some mechanism to provide glucose for these cells, even if that mechanism damaged or killed other cells; there is, after all, no point in having a healthy liver if your brain is dying.

Insulin resistance tries to preserve insulin-independent cells, regardless of the cost, by keeping our glucose levels from dropping too much. It works very well, and it helps most of us stay alive long enough to raise our children. The price we pay for the help we get from insulin resistance is that many of us will develop potbelly syndrome.

HOW INFECTIONS (AND OTHER STRESSES) CAUSE POTBELLY SYNDROME

There is always some cortisol present in the bloodstream, and it partially counteracts—*counterregulates* is the technical term—the activities of insulin. If infections or other stresses raise cortisol levels, then counterregulation increases and glucose levels rise.

Counterregulation raises glucose levels by slowing the movement of glucose into insulin-dependent cells and by facilitating the movement of glucose out of those same cells. The net result is an increase in the amount of glucose in the blood. The extra glucose can be used to help us cope with infections, missed meals, and other stressors. Counterregulation is not a sign of any kind of illness—it is a normal process that occurs throughout the day in everyone.

Insulin-dependent cells normally alternate between burning glucose and fat. As counterregulation increases, these cells burn less glucose and more fat. There is a net reduction in the amount of fuel burned, body temperature falls slightly, and there is a reduction in the amount of work that our cells can do. Counterregulated cells are partially deprived of proteins, so they have trouble repairing themselves. Counterregulation puts a strain on our insulin-dependent cells, but it does not injure them unless the strain is very severe or it persists for a long time. If we enjoy frequent recovery periods in which we are healthy, rested, and unstressed, cells that are strained will quickly repair themselves.

Insulin resistance. When we are under chronic stress, from infections or other causes, counterregulation becomes insulin resistance. Our metabolism is unbalanced, as shown in Figure 8.3. Our cells always have too much or too little of something, but they seldom have everything they need to stay healthy. They work poorly, and they make us feel mildly *dysphoric*, that is, we feel restless, anxious, uncomfortable. Physical activities are mildly unpleasant, and we tend to avoid unnecessary movements. If we walk anywhere, it is because we hope that walking is good for us. Truly healthy people enjoy walking.

When we feel dysphoric, we soon learn that eating carbohydrates, especially sugar, will make us feel better. After eating a doughnut or a candy bar, our glucose levels, which are already high, rise even higher for an hour or so. During this time, our insulin-dependent cells get more glucose and we feel better. Then our blood glucose drops and the dysphoria returns.

A craving for carbohydrates is not the same thing as hunger. Hunger

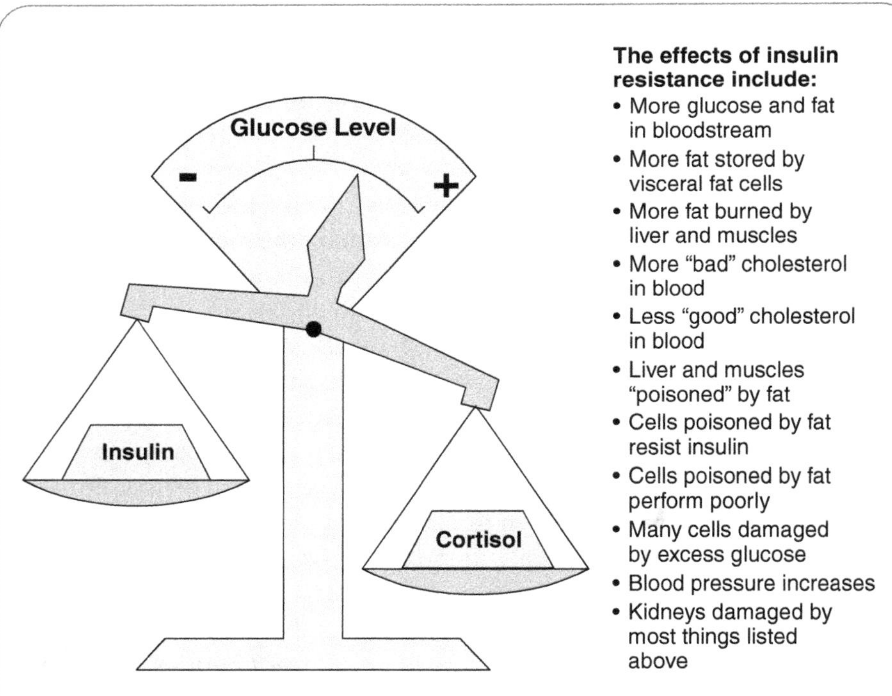

Figure 8.3. Insulin Resistance Develops When the Effects of Cortisol Overwhelm the Effects of Insulin

Cortisol counterregulates (opposes) many of the actions of insulin, causing insulin and glucose levels to rise. When counterregulation is severe or chronic, it is is called *insulin resistance.*

makes our stomachs hurt; the craving caused by insulin resistance is a more diffused feeling of discomfort. Carbohydrates can be highly addictive to people with insulin resistance, and many of us learn to avoid dysphoria by eating extra carbohydrates *before* we feel bad.

To stay active and function reasonably well, people with insulin resistance tend to keep their glucose levels high by avoiding exercise and eating carbohydrates. Their digestive systems produce more glucose than they can burn, and the unburned glucose is converted to fat.

Potbelly syndrome. In men and postmenopausal women, the excess fat tends to accumulate in visceral (stomach) fat cells. Fat also accumulates in liver and muscle cells, which are not supposed to store fat. Fat "poisons" liver and muscle cells and makes them more insulin resistant. This initiates a vicious cycle in which insulin resistance, by damaging our cells, makes us more insulin resistant. We now have Reaven's syndrome X, the first stage of potbelly syndrome. As years go by, we accumulate more of the disorders listed in Table 7.1 (page 72).

INFECTIONS AND INSULIN RESISTANCE

Insulin resistance is a normal part of every infection. People with the worst infections, such as those in septic shock, have such high levels of cortisol and insulin resistance that they may starve to death in a few days even though there is plenty of glucose in their blood.

What if we have a milder infection that lasts for days or weeks? While the infection lasts, glucose, insulin, and cortisol levels remain high. Fat piles up around our waist. Our muscle and liver cells are starved for glucose even though we are eating normally. Muscles become sore and weak, and they begin to melt away. Insulin resistance explains, at least in part, why athletes may need a year to fully recover from viral infections.[1,2]

What if we have a chronic infection such as AIDS or *C. pneumoniae*? The whole body is saturated with excess glucose, insulin, and cortisol for years, and dozens of things go wrong. Muscles and organs waste away while fat accumulates, and cholesterol plugs up our arteries. We feel rotten and we're too tired, too sick, and too depressed to exercise. We take stimulants to keep functioning, but the stimulants increase our cortisol burdens. If our joints hurt, or we have trouble breathing, our doctors give us cortisol-like medicines. We are now on a slippery slope that accelerates our progression to the advanced stages of potbelly syndrome.

HOW MUCH FOOD IS TOO MUCH?

Common sense tells us that people who are overweight "eat too much," but common sense is wrong. Most overweight people are insulin resistant, and people with insulin resistance generally eat just enough to get by.

The assumption that insulin-resistant people eat too much is based on the belief that there is a single, ideal amount of food for each person that will keep that person slender, healthy, and active. This belief is true for insulin-sensitive people, but it is completely wrong for insulin-resistant people. Insulin-resistant people have conflicting food needs, and they must decide which need they are going to satisfy. They must choose—and the choices are almost never consciously thought out—whether they want to:

- **Look like models**—People with insulin resistance can, with drugs, surgery, or an enormous effort, reduce their food intake until they look like fashion models. If they do so, they are likely to have numerous and serious health problems (Chapter 12).
- **Stay as healthy as possible**—There is probably an exact amount of food that each insulin-resistant person should eat to optimize her health. No one knows exactly how much food that is, but it appears to be more than models eat, and it may not be enough food to allow her to function well. This is a good choice for people who can visit a spa in Palm Springs when things get rough.
- **Function reasonably well**—To function well in a busy, stressful world, insulin-resistant people must eat more food, especially carbohydrates, than they can burn. Without the extra food, they become dysphoric, tired, and cranky. With the extra food, they gain weight and become more insulin resistant.

The three choices available to people with insulin resistance are pretty grim. If they eat enough to stay busy, they are eating too much to stay slim or healthy. Regardless of which choice they make, insulin-resistant people do not, in any broad, general sense, "eat too much."

SUMMARY

Cortisol-induced counterregulation is a normal response to stress. It raises glucose levels to ensure the continued functioning of brain cells and other insulin-independent cells. Counterregulation imposes strains on liver and muscle cells, but they are not harmed unless the counterregulation progresses to insulin resistance.

Insulin resistance becomes self-sustaining, to some extent, by damaging cells in ways that make them more insulin resistant. Furthermore, insulin resistance makes us crave carbohydrates, and it punishes us with dysphoria if we don't eat them. The extra carbohydrates make us gain weight, and the extra weight increases our dysphoria every time we look in a mirror.

Cortisol-induced insulin resistance is the mechanism by which middle-path germs cause potbelly syndrome.

RECOMMENDED READING

Insulin resistance is the central element of all versions of the dysmetabolic syndrome X. That being the case, you might be interested in the following books, even though none of them deal with germs or cortisol.

Syndrome X: Managing Insulin Resistance, by Deborah S. Romaine and Jennifer Marks, M.D. (HarperTorch, 2000).

This excellent book contains a chapter on polycystic ovarian syndrome (PCOS), a condition that resembles Cushing's syndrome in some ways.

Syndrome X: Overcoming the Silent Killer That Can Give You a Heart Attack, by Gerald Reaven, M.D., Terry Kristen Strom, M.B.A., and Barry Fox, Ph.D. (Simon and Schuster, 2000).

Dr. Reaven coined the term "Syndrome X" and it is his definition of it that we used when defining the stages of hypercortisolism. This is an excellent book.

Syndrome X: The Complete Nutritional Program to Prevent and Reverse Insulin Resistance, by Jack Challem, Burt Berkson, M.D., and Melissa Diane Smith (Wiley, 2000).

This book has a great deal of valuable information on nonmedical methods of dealing with Syndrome X.

REFERENCES

Epigraph: Challem J, Berkson B, and Smith MD. *Syndrome X: The Complete Nutritional Program to Prevent and Reverse Insulin Resistance.* New York: Wiley, 2000.

1. Jakeman P. A longitudinal study of exercise metabolism during recovery from viral illness. *Br J Sports Med.* 1993 Sep;27(3):157–161.

2. Maffulli N, Testa V, and Capasso G. Post-viral fatigue syndrome. A longitudinal assessment in varsity athletes. *J Sports Med Phys Fitness* 1993 Dec;33(4): 392–399.

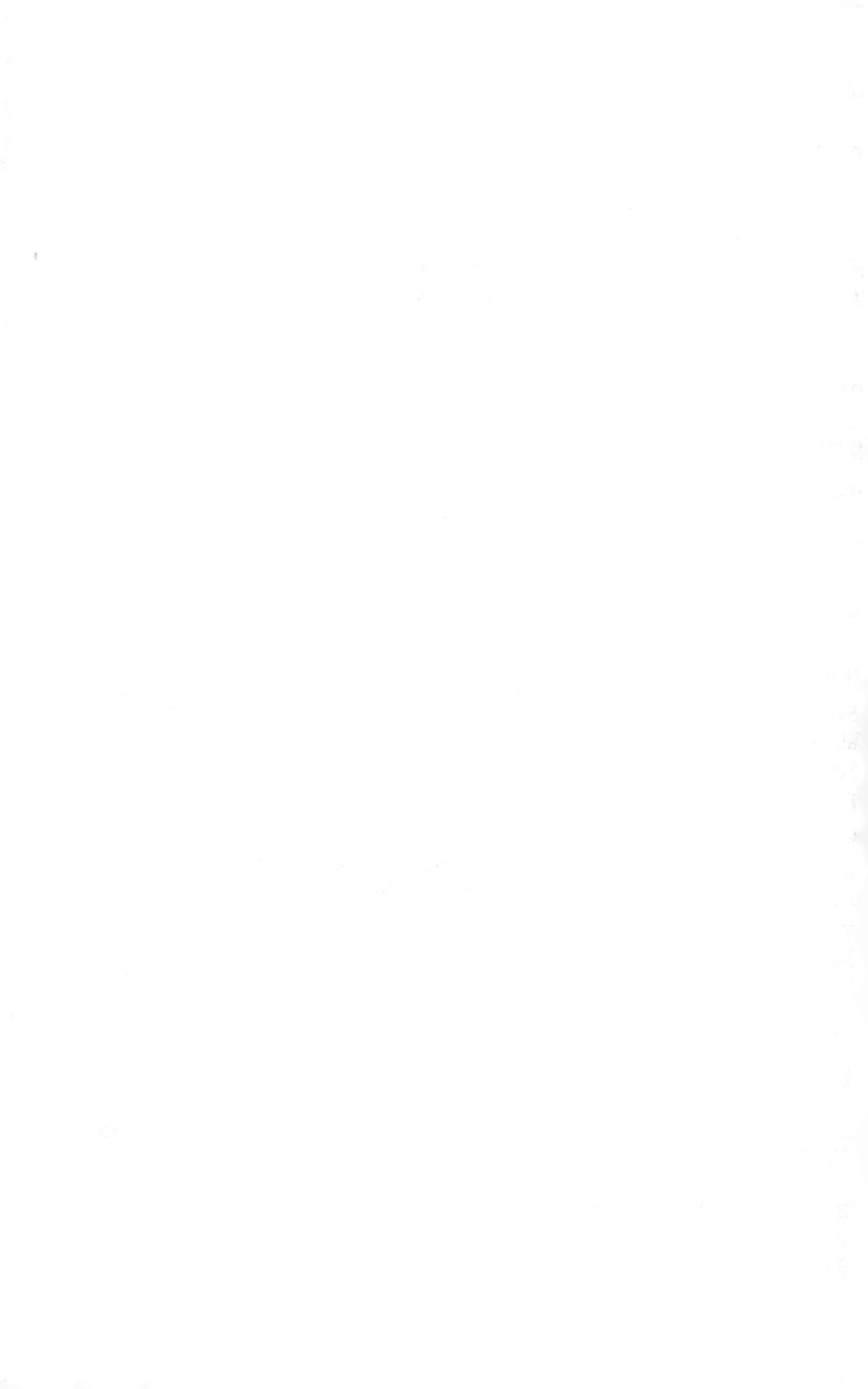

9

How Stress Affects Fat Storage

Living organisms, including people, are merely tubes which put things in at one end and let them out at the other, which both keeps them doing it and in the long run wears them out. . . . At the input end they develop ganglia of nerves called brains, with eyes and ears, so that they can more easily scrounge around for things to swallow. . . . All this seems marvelously futile, and yet, when you begin to think about it, it begins to seem more marvelous than futile. Indeed, it seems extremely odd.

—ALAN W. WATTS, *THE BOOK ON THE TABOO AGAINST KNOWING WHO YOU ARE*

Getting enough to eat is the oldest and most fundamental activity of life, older than sleep, older than sex, older even than breathing. Our ancestors were a thousand times more likely to die from starvation than from overeating. Despite the odds, every one of our ancestors avoided starvation long enough to reach the age of reproduction. Consequently, we are really good at finding and storing food.

Just as Mother Nature prefers high blood pressure to low, and high blood sugar to low, she also prefers for us to be overweight rather than underweight, and she has provided us with a very efficient fat-storage system. This chapter discusses some of the factors that control fat storage, with an emphasis on the role of stress in making us store extra fat.

LIPOSTATS AND SET POINTS

Before our ancestors developed pottery and basketry, the only way they could store food was to eat as much as they could and let some of it turn into fat. When food was scarce again, fat was burned for fuel. The constant weight cycling was bad for their health, but it was not as bad as starvation, so the ability to store fat efficiently had a high survival value.

There was an upper limit to how much fat our ancestors could store, however. If they stored too much, they would be slow on their feet, and predators would kill them. To stay plump, but not too fat, our ancestors evolved a fat-regulating system—a *lipostat*—to control the amount of fat they stored when food was abundant, and the amount they burned when food was scarce.

The Lipostat Theory Is Still Under Construction

There is wide acceptance of the idea that lipostats exist, but there is no consensus, in 2005, on how they work. The description presented here is an extremely simplified "best guess." This guess explains some of the mysteries of weight control, and it fits the information available in 2005 reasonably well, but it is not as firmly rooted in research as the other material in this book.

Lipostats work a little like the thermostats that control the temperature in your house. Both systems work by comparing *set point* values with actual values. You select a set point temperature by turning a knob. The thermostat compares the set point temperature with the actual temperature, and then "decides" what to do. If the actual temperature is lower than the set point temperature, then the thermostat turns the furnace on and heats the room until the set point and actual temperatures match.

The two values compared by a lipostat appear to be stress level and *leptin* level.

The lipostat uses your stress level to "estimate" how much fat you should be storing to cope with the stresses in your life. Since the amount of fat you store is closely related to your weight, we can say that the lipostat uses your stress level to estimate how much you should weigh. We can call this hypothetical weight your *fat-storage set point* (FSSP) *weight.*

Leptin is a hormone produced by fat cells, and leptin levels are proportional to the amount of fat that is stored, so leptin levels are roughly proportional to your actual weight.

To say that lipostats compare stress levels with leptin levels is almost the same thing as saying that lipostats compare FSSP weights with actual weights.

If your actual weight is more than your FSSP weight, the lipostat initiates physiological and psychological changes that will lower your cortisol level, interfere with fat storage, raise your body temperature, and make you more active. You will lose an ounce or two every day until your actual weight matches your FSSP weight.

If your actual weight is less than your FSSP weight, the lipostat initiates changes that will raise your cortisol level, facilitate fat storage, lower your body temperature, and make you less active. You will gain an ounce or two every day until your actual weight matches your FSSP weight. Figure 9.1 illustrates the interaction of FSSP weight and actual weight.

The behavior of the proposed lipostat is very similar to that of the hypothalamic-pituitary-adrenal (HPA) axis which controls cortisol levels. This is not a coincidence. The lipostat and HPA axis share the same organs and parts of the brain, and they involve many of the same cytokines and hormones. Eventually, when we understand these topics better, I suspect that we will find that controlling fat storage is simply a collateral duty of the HPA axis.

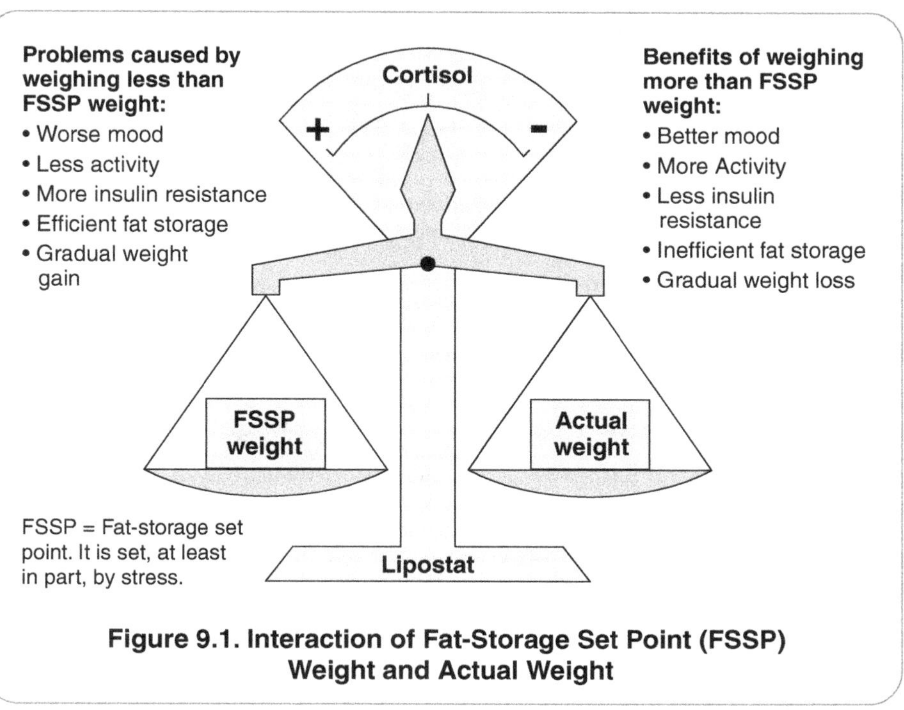

Figure 9.1. Interaction of Fat-Storage Set Point (FSSP) Weight and Actual Weight

RATCHETING YOUR WEIGHT UP

When you tighten a nut with a ratchet wrench, you rotate the wrench clockwise for a fraction of a turn, then rotate it back counterclockwise. Each time you repeat these two motions, the nut is turned—ratcheted—clockwise and becomes tighter. There is a similar effect involved in trying to lose weight. As we try to lose weight, our weight goes up and down, but it almost always goes up a little more than it went down. The result is that our weight is slowly ratcheted upward.

If we accept the fairly obvious notion that dieting is stressful, the lipostat model explains why dieting ratchets our weight up a little more with each loss-gain cycle. To illustrate how this happens, let's try another thought experiment.

Imagine a handsome young fellow named Clem whose weight is creeping up two or three pounds a year. He feels fine, but he doesn't like the way he looks. When his FSSP weight and his actual weight reach 225, he clamps his jaws shut and vows to lose 25 pounds. Here is what is likely to happen:

- Clem easily drops his actual weight down to 210. He feels okay at first because the difference between his actual weight and his FSSP weight is only 15 pounds.
- Clem's hypothalamus—a key part of the lipostat—understands famines, but not diets. When it notices that Clem is losing weight, the hypothalamus decides that a famine is coming and it raises his FSSP weight to 250 pounds.
- The hypothalamus triggers the release of extra cortisol to help Clem raise his actual weight closer to his new FSSP weight.
- The extra cortisol increases Clem's insulin resistance and damages cells throughout his body. The damaged cells make him feel rotten. Carbohydrates, especially sugar, make him feel better temporarily, and Clem develops an overpowering urge to eat more carbohydrates.
- Despite heroic efforts, Clem's weight "ratchets" back up to 225 in a few months. The problem now is that his actual weight is 25 pounds below his new FSSP weight.
- Clem has to struggle mightily just to stay at the weight he was comfortable at a few months before.
- The more Clem diets, the higher his FSSP weight climbs. His actual weight goes up and down, but it always ratchets up more than down.

Now, instead of gaining 2 or 3 pounds a year, he gains 5 or 10. Instead of being comfortable and healthy at 225, he will be miserable and insulin resistant at 240, 250, and so on.

- At last, Clem acknowledges defeat and stops trying to lose weight. His weight stabilizes at about 275, and he feels fine, except when he looks in a mirror.
- Now that Clem's FSSP and actual weights match, his cortisol level and insulin resistance levels are lower than when he was struggling to keep his weight down.

Clem was trying to lose weight without first lowering his FSSP weight. He was doomed to failure, but he is not alone because most people who try to lose weight fail, and they fail for similar reasons. We will join Clem for another attempt at losing weight in Chapter 12, but here I want to show you what happens to people who try to *raise* their actual weights above their FSSP weights.

OVERFEEDING EXPERIMENTS AND FAT RESISTANCE

Everyone knows fat-resistant people who, like my friend Slim, can eat huge quantities of food and never grow fat. When I go to dinner with people like Slim, they are deciding whether to have sirloin or filet while I'm deciding whether to have iceberg or romaine. It would be easy to hate these people, but the ones I know are invariably cheerful and likable. (Are they cheerful because they eat so much, or do they metabolize their food well because they're cheerful? If you figure this out, let me know.)

Slim would not be envied in Cameroon, where obesity is seen as a sign of virility, strength, and prestige. In the Cameroonian *guru walla* ceremony, young men are fed prodigious amounts of food for months to make them fat. They are discouraged from exercising, and typically gain about 35 pounds.[1] Since we are taught from childhood that eating too much is bad for us, we would expect something awful to happen to these young men, but they survive their ordeal in good health and fine spirits. The *guru walla* celebrants return to their normal weights, without dieting or joining a gym, in about three years.

Closer to home, three researchers from the Mayo Clinic studied the effects of intentional overfeeding on sixteen slender, sedentary subjects. The subjects were studied for two weeks to determine how many calories they needed every day to maintain their weight. Then they were given an extra 1,000 calories a day for eight weeks (that's 56,000 extra calories). Overfeeding made the subjects more active, so they only gained about half of the weight we would have expected; they gained 5.26 pounds of fat and 5.17 pounds of nonfat mass.[2] The researchers described the additional activity as: ". . . physical activities other than volitional exercise, such as the activities of daily living, fidgeting, spontaneous muscle contraction, and maintaining posture when not recumbent."[3]

Their leptin increased by 61 percent, so it is not too surprising that the subjects of this high-tech *guru walla* returned to their normal weights within two weeks.

The most interesting thing about this experiment, from the standpoint of anyone trying to lose weight, is that there was a wide range of fat resistance in the subjects. The most fat-resistant subject gained less than a pound of fat, while the least fat-resistant gained 9.3 pounds.

The most fat-resistant subjects were the most active, but what made them more active than their peers? Were they the healthiest? The most cheerful? We'll never know because questions like these were beyond the scope of the Mayo Clinic study. Research is expensive, and the most interesting questions often sound frivolous to the people paying for the research.

In the previous chapter, I explained how insulin resistance leads to weight gain, but most health professionals believe that the opposite is true. If obesity does cause insulin resistance, then we would expect people who are overfed to become more insulin resistant, but that is not the case. Researchers in Indianapolis overfed six slender, active, young adults for several weeks. At the end of this period, the subjects had gained an average of 9.7 pounds and their leptin level had risen 68 percent.[4] Five of the six subjects became *less* insulin resistant!

These few studies, though small, strongly support the set point theory, and they show that raising our weight above our set point is, in the long run, as difficult as lowering our weight below it. Just as most dieters regain any weight they lose, the overfed subjects in these experiments quickly lost the weight they gained.

SUMMARY

The lipostat monitors our stress levels and "calculates" a fat-storage set point (FSSP) weight. Our actual weight tends to rise or fall, as necessary, to match our FSSP weight.

Neither willpower nor wishing will reduce our FSSP weight. We can, with enough willpower, force our actual weight to stay below our FSSP weight, but we will experience both physiological and psychological problems in the process. Forcing our actual weight down is stressful, and the extra stress raises our FSSP weight. Since the lipostat usually wins in the long run, trying to force our weight down accelerates the rate at which our weight goes up.

The stresses that establish our FSSP weights can be of any kind, but the most important are those caused by middle-path germs. Ordinary, daily stresses tend to come and go, and weight gain caused by daily stresses will disappear when the stresses disappear. Chronic infections almost never disappear, and they become more numerous as we get older, so we tend to get heavier as we get older.

I believe that the only safe way for most of us to lose weight is to reduce our FSSP weight by reducing stress. When that is done, we can just relax and our actual weight will drop until it matches the new FSSP weight. Chapters 15 through 20 discuss ways of reducing stress.

RECOMMENDED RESOURCE

Chuck Forsberg is a computer wizard who maintains a website with interesting information about fat. The URL is: www.omen.com/adipos.html.

REFERENCES

Epigraph: Watts, Alan W. *The Book: On the Taboo Against Knowing Who You Are.* New York, NY: Collier Books, 1966.

1. Pasquet P, Brigant L, Froment A, et al. Massive overfeeding and energy balance in men: The *Guru Walla* model. *Am J Clin Nutr* 1992 Sep;56(3):483–490.

2. Levine JA, Eberhardt NL, and Jensen MD. Leptin responses to overfeeding: Relationship with body fat and nonexercise activity thermogenesis. *J Clin Endocrinol Metab* 1999 Aug;84(8):2751–2754.

3. Levine JA, Eberhardt NL, and Jensen MD. Role of nonexercise activity thermogenesis in resistance to fat gain in humans. *Science* 1999 Jan 8;283(5399):212–224.

4. Ohannesian JP, Marco CC, Najm PS, et al. Small weight gain is not associated with development of insulin resistance in healthy, physically active individuals. *Horm Metab Res* 1999 May;31(5):323–325.

10

How Stress Affects Appetite

Overweight individuals are often derided for their assertion, "But I eat like a bird." It is usually taken for granted that they are more or less knowingly lying. Another assumption, hardly more generous, is that they do not possess the wit to observe and judge the quantity of food that they consume. Is it not conceivable that these—the too easily and too frequently condemned—are, in terms of the urgent appetites which drive them, heroes of rigorous self-mastery?

—JEAN MAYER, *OVERWEIGHT: CAUSES, COST, AND CONTROL*, 1968

A good appetite was so important to the survival of our ancestors that they evolved an extremely complex system, called an *appestat,* to ensure that they would eat heartily when food was abundant, but not eat too much. To make this system easier to understand, we will break it into four subsystems, as follows:

- The stress-leptin subsystem, which makes us hungry when our actual weight drops below a set point weight.
- The glucose (blood sugar) subsystem, which makes us hungry when our glucose level drops below a set point.
- The ghrelin subsystem, which makes us hungry before meals.
- The empty-stomach subsystem, which makes us hungry when our stomach is empty.

All four subsystems are designed to make us hungry—none of them are designed to make us feel satiated (the opposite of hungry). When one of these subsystems "decides" we have had enough to eat, it stops contributing to our feelings of hunger. We never feel completely satiated, however, until all four subsystems simultaneously agree that we have had enough to eat.

If there is an error in the operation of an appestat subsystem, the error will almost always make us hungrier than we should be. Cases where all four subsystems err in such a way as to prevent us from feeling hunger, as in the case of anorexia nervosa, are very rare.

The appestat subsystems use some of the same organs, hormones, and parts of the brain that the HPA axis uses to control cortisol. Figure 10.1 shows how some of those factors complement or oppose each other to make us feel hunger or satiety. This chapter will describe the appestat subsystems very briefly and review some interesting studies of appetite and eating behavior.

THE STRESS-LEPTIN SUBSYSTEM

The stress-leptin subsystem is similar to the lipostat described in the previous chapter. It establishes an *appetite set point (ASP) weight* that may or may not be

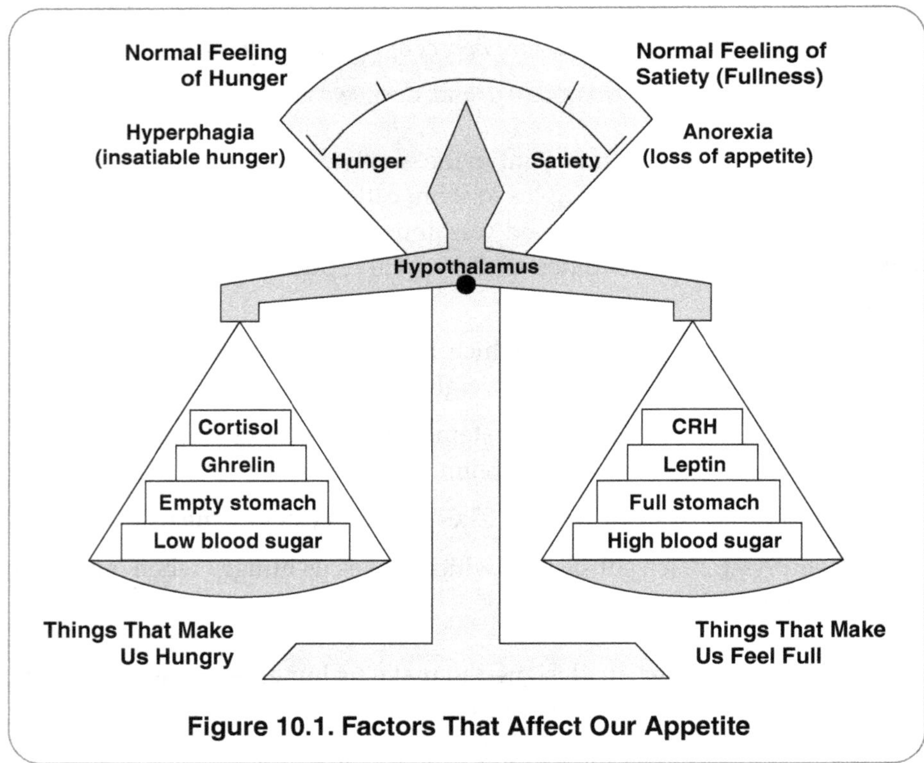

Figure 10.1. Factors That Affect Our Appetite

the same thing as the fat-storage set point (FSSP) weight discussed in the last chapter. When our actual weight is below the ASP weight, the hypothalamus releases *corticotropin-releasing hormone* (CRH), which triggers the release of *adrenocorticotropic* hormone, which, in turn, triggers the release of cortisol. CRH suppresses appetite and cortisol stimulates it.[1] Because of the opposing effects of these two hormones, our response to stress is an initial loss of appetite followed by an increase of appetite. Chronic stresses lead to chronic increases in our appetite.

When our actual weight is less than our ASP weight, the extra cortisol keeps us hungry night and day until our actual weight rises to match our ASP weight.

THE GLUCOSE SUBSYSTEM

In Chapter 8 we saw that low glucose can trigger the release of cortisol. When this happens, the extra cortisol increases counterregulation to raise blood sugar quickly. The extra cortisol also makes us hungry for carbohydrates, since they raise our glucose levels rapidly.

THE GHRELIN SUBSYSTEM

Ghrelin is a hormone produced in the stomach, and it stimulates our appetites before meals. Here is a short summary of its known and suspected activities:

- Ghrelin rises before meals and falls after we eat.
- Ghrelin rises when we lose weight by dieting.
- Ghrelin appears to stimulate cortisol production.
- Ghrelin production—and hence appetite—may be increased by some infections, and reduced by others.

Ghrelin is probably a very important hormone, but it was only discovered a few years ago, and we don't know much about it yet.

THE EMPTY-STOMACH SUBSYSTEM

The stomach and the hypothalamus are connected to each other by nerves running in both directions. When the stomach is empty, nerve impulses from the stomach travel to the hypothalamus. If the hypothalamus decides that it is time to eat, it sends hunger signals that make the stomach cramp. The cramps are painful, and they remind us to eat. After we eat something, the stomach sends not-empty signals to the hypothalamus. The hypothalamus weighs all of its information, including the not-empty signals, and decides whether or not to continue giving us hunger pains.

Dieters often try to fool the hypothalamus, and reduce the number of calories they consume, by filling their stomachs with bulky, low-calorie food. This never works for more than a few days because the hypothalamus, primitive as it is, soon learns to ignore the not-empty signals from a stomach full of lettuce and celery. When this happens, the hypothalamus can make us feel hungry even when we are stuffed, and we tend to eat too often and too much.

It's very hard to fool Mother Nature.

STRESS-RESISTANCE AND APPETITE

The ability to resist stress varies greatly from person to person. A recent study showed that stress-resistant subjects ate less than stress-sensitive subjects after experiencing similar stresses. Elissa Epel and colleagues, from the University of California at San Francisco, studied the effect of stress on fifty-nine healthy women. She and her colleagues subjected the women, one at a time, to a mildly stressful situation and then left them in a comfortable room with a basket containing four snacks. The women, who did not know that the study was about eating, were invited to eat as many of the snacks as they wished. There were four kinds of snacks: high-fat and sweet; high-fat and salty; low-fat and sweet; and low-fat and salty.

Three days later, the women had a nonstressful session at the same laboratory and were again left in the comfortable room with the basket of snacks.

During both visits, the women's salivary cortisol levels were checked several times, and the women were divided into two groups on the basis of their cortisol levels. The "low cortisol reactors" were presumably more stress resistant than the "high cortisol reactors." After each woman left the laboratory, Dr. Epel's researchers counted the number of snacks she had eaten. The results of the study are summarized in Table 10.1.[2]

The stress these women experienced was mild and of short duration. Still, in the hour following the stress, the women whose cortisol levels rose the most consumed almost twice as many calories as the women with the smallest increase in cortisol. This was a small study, and the subjects were

TABLE 10.1. INTERACTION OF STRESS, CORTISOL, AND APPETITE

Subjects	Stressful Session	Relaxed Session
Low cortisol reactors		Ate more total snacks.
High cortisol reactors	Ate nearly twice as many calories. Ate more high-fat snacks. Ate more high-fat, sweet snacks. Mood worse than low reactors.	Ate more sweet snacks.

only studied for a short time, but I can't help wondering what will happen to these stress-sensitive women in the future. If they live happy, low-stress lives, they may be alright. But what will happen to them if they are exposed to the normal stresses of a busy life for thirty or forty years? If Dr. Epel does a follow-up study, I predict that the stress-resistant women will be thinner, healthier, and happier than the stress-sensitive women.

Chapter 19 discusses ways of increasing our stress resistance.

PERPETUAL HUNGER

The authors of diet books imply that once you lose weight by their method you will be able to keep the weight off effortlessly. Not so. Unless you have lowered your appetite set point weight, you will be hungry night and day until you return to your previous weight.

People on diets are perpetually hungry because their cortisol levels are perpetually elevated. Researchers from Laval University in Quebec measured how hungry their subjects were before breakfast. Then the subjects began a strict fifteen-week diet (phase 1). At the end of this phase, the subjects' prebreakfast hunger was measured again. Guess what—after fifteen weeks of calorie restriction, the subjects were hungrier than when they began.[3] Phase 2 consisted of a follow-up program with exercise and a low-fat diet. At the end of phase 2, the subjects' pre-breakfast hunger was even greater than it had been after phase 1. After analyzing their results, these researchers concluded:

> These results suggest that weight loss is accompanied by an increase of baseline appetite in both men and women and that the most consistent predictor of these changes in appetite seems to be changes in fasting plasma cortisol.[4]

FOOLS FOR FOOD

Can the hormones that control our appetites make fools out of us? I think so. For years I took long walks around my neighborhood, and these walks almost always led me to greasy, sugary carbohydrates. I rationalized each trip to my local doughnut shop with some variation on the thought that I deserved a treat after my heroic efforts to lose weight. Every morning, the urge for a maple bar would overpower my sixty-year-old brain just the way my urge for, well, let's skip her name, had overpowered my twenty-year-old brain.

We have all read how Dr. Pavlov was able to shape the behavior of dogs by rewarding them for behaviors he wanted. I think that Mother Nature shapes our thought processes by hormonal rewards and punishments. The thought processes that Mother Nature wants us to develop are appropriate for young people living in a tribe of hunter-gatherers, but they are inappropriate for an old guy living near a doughnut shop.

When our evolutionary history is considered, consciously trying to lose weight has to be seen as one of the most unnatural acts that a young hunter-gatherer could perform. Is it any wonder that Mother Nature tries to prevent such perverse behavior, even in old people who are seriously overweight?

The effects that hormones have on our thought processes are obvious once you start looking for them, but lots of things that are obvious are not true. I couldn't find any firm scientific support for my food-makes-us-foolish theory, but I did find a couple of interesting studies.

We know that cortisol and leptin control fat storage and appetite. Can they affect our behavior? Canadian researchers allowed rats access to food for two hours a day. They found that skinny rats—which presumably had lower leptin levels—hoarded more food than fat ones did.[5] Does our cortisol-leptin balance affect our food choices in the supermarket as well as at the table? Does it affect our decisions about exercising? What other life decisions might be influenced by cortisol and/or leptin?

Another study found that overweight women with type 2 diabetes underreported how much they ate by about 800 calories per day. The more obese these women were, the more likely they were to underreport the food they ate.[6] Were these women consciously lying? No, it appears that they believed their reports. This brings up the interesting possibility that hormones may shape both our behaviors and our recollections of those behaviors. This is another topic that begs for more research. Until such research is done, we need to monitor our own cognitive processes and see how we might be tricking ourselves into eating too much.

SUMMARY

The U.S. National Institute of Diabetes and Digestive and Kidney Diseases summarized the importance of set points:

> Treatments for obesity are notoriously ineffective when measured by the yardstick of success in the maintenance of reduced body weight. An understanding of the nature of the components for the set point system would provide physiologic and pharmacological tools for the successful treatment of obesity and diabetes.[7]

In plainer English, they are saying that current methods of losing weight don't work, but there might be a way of getting people to lose weight by lowering their set points. As we have seen, set point weights appear to be determined by stress, and the best way to lower them is to reduce our stress levels, a topic that will be explored in Chapters 15 through 20.

RECOMMENDED READING

Fight Fat after Forty, by Pamela Peeke (Viking, 2000).

Dr. Peeke is an expert on stress, hormones, and obesity. Her book is well written and easy to read.

REFERENCES

Epigraph: Mayer, Jean. *Overweight: Causes, Cost, and Control.* Englewood Cliffs, NJ: Prentice-Hall, Collier Books, 1968, p. 5.

1. Peeke, Pamela. *Fight Fat After Forty.* New York, NY: Viking, 2000, p. 107.

2. Epel E, Lapidus R, McEwen B, et al. Stress may add bite to appetite in women: A laboratory study of stress-induced cortisol and eating behavior. *Psychoneuroendocrinology* 2001 Jan;26(1):37–49.

3. Doucet E, Imbeault P, St-Pierre S, et al. Appetite after weight loss by energy restriction and a low-fat diet-exercise follow-up. *Int J Obes Relat Metab Disord* 2000 Jul;24(7):906–914.

4. Ibid. p. 906.

5. Cabanac M and Gosselin C. Ponderostat: Hoarding behavior satisfies the condition for a lipostat in the rat. *Appetite* 1996 Dec;27(3):251–261.

6. Mann, Denise. Most Overweight Women Have Inaccurate Memories of Meal Size; Do You Know What You Ate Last Summer? WebMD;July 2, 2001.

7. FY 1999 Program Plan Research Progress Reviews. Division of Digestive Diseases and Nutrition, National Institute of Diabetes and Digestive and Kidney Diseases, p. 25.

11

Cortisol, Infections, and Potbellies

I would sell my soul to the devil to be one of those girls who can eat nine sausages for breakfast, a huge plate of eggs and never gain a pound. I might make a pact with Satan to get a better metabolic rate.

—ELIZABETH HURLEY, BRITISH ACTRESS

Does excess cortisol really cause potbellies? Absolutely. When people take cortisol-like medicines, they often develop potbellies within a few months. When someone develops a tumor that stimulates cortisol production, the first visible sign of it will be a potbelly. People with AIDS often develop high cortisol levels and potbellies even while their muscles waste away. Children starved until their arms are no bigger around than your thumb will often have high cortisol levels and potbellies. Cortisol indisputably causes potbellies.

Yet, when researchers weigh a group of people and measure their cortisol levels, the links between cortisol and obesity can be confusing and contradictory.[1,2] These conflicting research results are caused by the following factors:

- The effects of cortisol on weight vary with the sex, race, age, education, and social status of the people being studied.
- Some researchers measure blood and saliva cortisol levels, which are only loosely associated with weight, while others measure urinary cortisol levels, which are more closely associated with weight.
- Some researchers measure only morning cortisol levels, so they fail to detect the higher evening cortisol levels that are associated with potbellies.

- Some researchers measure diffuse obesity, which is not closely linked to cortisol, while others measure abdominal obesity, which is closely linked to cortisol.

When you look at hundreds of studies, and make allowances for who is being studied, and how the studies are being done, it is clear that excess cortisol is a major cause of obesity. This chapter will discuss cortisol's role in causing obesity, and we will begin by comparing apples and pears.

APPLES VERSUS PEARS

Overweight men tend to have well-defined potbellies, and overweight women tend to have their extra pounds diffused over their bodies, with a lot of it settling on their hips and thighs. Years ago, someone named these patterns of fat distribution "apple shaped" and "pear shaped." It takes a lot of imagination to see people as apples or pears, but the terms have stuck, so we will use them here.

We have several kinds of fat cells, and they are clustered together in fat depots scattered around the body. In healthy, normal-weight people, most of their fat depots have a little fat in them at all times.

As we saw in Chapters 8 and 9, fat storage is controlled by hormones. Insulin tends to make all fat cells store more fat, and glucagon tends to make all fat cells release fat. Cortisol produces apple-shaped people by accelerating the storage of fat in abdominal fat depots. The "female" hormones estrogen and progesterone appear to block some of the effects of cortisol, so young women are not as likely as men to have potbellies. After menopause, when estrogen and progesterone levels fall, women are as likely as men to develop potbellies.

There are probably hormones that produce pear-shaped people, but they have not been identified yet.

There are a few other hormones that affect our shape. Thyroid hormones accelerate our metabolism and help us burn fat, and the "male" hormone testosterone helps build muscles that help to burn fat. When these hormones are low, we develop a soft layer of fat that is diffused over most of the body. Cortisol may contribute to diffused obesity because it suppresses thyroid hormones and testosterone.

Most of the illnesses and disorders associated with obesity are only associated with potbellies, and pear-shaped people, no matter how unhappy they may be with the way they look, do not have as many health problems as apple-shaped people.

How do you know if you are an apple or a pear? If a look in the mirror doesn't tell you, then calculate your waist-to-hip ratio, or, easier yet, just measure your waist.

Waist-to-hip ratio (WHR). To find your WHR, measure your waist and hips. Divide the waist measurement by the hip measurement. A woman with a 35-inch waist and 46-inch hips, for example, would have a WHR of 0.76. Women with WHRs more than 0.8, and men with WHRs more than 1.0, are considered "apples" and they are at greater risk for heart attacks and strokes than people with smaller WHRs. Finnish researchers found that the people with the highest WHRs had the worst symptoms of Reaven's syndrome X.[3]

Waist size versus WHR. WHR calculations give the obesity problem a nice scientific air, but some researchers believe that the only measurement that really matters—from a health standpoint—is your waist size.

If you are a woman and your waist measures more than thirty-five inches, or if you are a man and your waist measures more than forty inches, you are more likely to develop heart disease, high blood pressure, diabetes, cancer, and all of the other diseases and disorders linked to obesity.[4]

Dr. Mårin describes an improvement on the waist-size measurement in Chapter 16. It's called the abdominal sagittal diameter (ASD) measurement.

DISORDERS BLAMED ON OBESITY

Cause and effect are often difficult to identify when studying chronic illnesses. Below are brief discussions of several common disorders. In some cases, the disorder and the obesity are both caused by excess cortisol. In other cases, such as breathing problems, the disorder causes hypercortisolism, and the hypercortisolism causes the obesity.

Breathing problems. We assume that obese people are short-winded because they must work harder to carry their extra weight. That is probably true, but it turns out that obese people also have lower lung capacities, and their reduced lung capacity may have made them obese.

If you grab a handful of skin around your waist, the thickness of the skinfold is a good indication of how much of your body is fat. Australian researchers found that the lung capacities of their subjects decreased as their skinfold thickness increased.[5]

Obese people are more likely than normal-weight people to suffer from both chronic obstructive pulmonary disease (COPD) and adult-onset asthma. It has been assumed for years that obesity causes these breathing problems, but it is more plausible to believe that the breathing problems caused the obesity. This is because reduced lung capacity, from any cause, results in chronic hypoxia—an oxygen deficiency in the body's tissues. Hypoxia stimulates cortisol production, which then leads to obesity.

Cancer. Obesity, especially the abdominal type, is associated with an increased mortality from cancer. Obese men are more likely than nonobese men to die from cancer of the colon, rectum, and prostate. Obese women are more likely than nonobese women to die from cancer of the gallbladder, breast, uterus, cervix, and ovaries.[6] It may be cortisol, not obesity, that causes obese people to be more cancer-prone. Cortisol suppresses the immune system, and obese people tend to have elevated cortisol levels and weakened immune systems. The weakened immune system might be unable to kill cancerous cells.

Even if cortisol inhibits the immune system's ability to kill cancer cells, this doesn't mean that lowering your cortisol level will help you fight cancer. Cortisol inhibits cell growth, and it may suppress the growth of some cancer cells. If you have cancer, be sure to talk to your doctor before making any direct attempt to reduce your cortisol levels.

Cardiovascular risk. Everyone knows that obese people are at a greater risk for cardiovascular problems, but it is also true that people with cardiovascular problems are at greater risk for obesity. Autopsy studies show that cardiovascular problems develop in most people long before obesity does. This fact suggests that heart disease is more likely to cause obesity than obesity is to cause heart disease.

Cataracts. A few years ago, researchers from Harvard discovered that people with large WHRs were more likely to develop cataracts.[7] There is no reason to believe that a large waist causes cataracts, but there are good reasons to believe that excess cortisol causes both cataracts and large waists. When researchers want their laboratory rats to develop cataracts, they treat them with cortisol.

Hypertension. One of the interesting phenomena associated with obesity is that a small drop in weight of as little as 5 percent can lower blood pressure and reduce diabetic problems noticeably.[8] This is usually taken as evidence that obesity caused the blood pressure and diabetes in the first place. Another plausible explanation is that some positive lifestyle change reduced cortisol levels, and weight, blood pressure, and diabetic symptoms improved as a result of the drop in cortisol.

On the other hand, fat cells produce cortisol, leptin, and angiotensin II, three hormones that raise blood pressure, so obesity does contribute to hypertension.

Immunodeficiency. When a person is given a vaccination for some germ X, he or she should develop antibodies against germ X. A failure to develop the antibodies indicates an immune problem. When civil service workers from Connecticut were vaccinated against the hepatitis B virus, the extremely obese workers were thirteen times as likely as their coworkers not to develop antibodies.[9] The inability to develop antibodies to germs is, like obesity, another symptom of excess cortisol.

Night-eating syndrome (NES). Do you get the "munchies" in the middle of the night? This urge to eat at night is closely linked to obesity, and people afflicted with it experience anorexia (loss of appetite) in the mornings and hyperphagia (great hunger) in the evenings. People with NES also suffer from insomnia; researchers from Norway found that people with NES woke up twelve times as often as the control subjects. Half of their awakenings were associated with eating. The people with NES had much higher cortisol levels than the controls did.[10] It appears that cortisol causes NES, and NES contributes to obesity.

Sleep apnea. Obese people are prone to suffer from sleep apnea, a condition in which they stop breathing for short periods throughout the night. The resulting hypoxia is very stressful and it raises cortisol levels. It has been assumed that obesity causes sleep apnea, but researchers from Kyoto, Japan, found that treating sleep apnea for six months resulted in a 23 percent reduction in the abdominal fat of their test subjects.[11] This suggests that sleep apnea causes obesity—the exact reverse of what conventional wisdom would have us believe.

Strokes. Obesity has been linked to strokes and other cerebrovascular problems. Strokes are also linked to *Chlamydophila pneumoniae* infections and excess cortisol.

GERMS LINKED TO OBESITY

Most infections cause weight loss, but there is a small but growing body of research showing that some germs make people and animals gain weight. A few of these germs are discussed below.

Adenovirus (type SMAM-1). There are many kinds of adenoviruses, and some of them infect humans. They seldom make humans seriously ill, but they often kill pets, wildlife, and farm animals. Chickens infected with the SMAM-1 strain of adenovirus develop large amounts of fat around their abdomens. Unexpectedly, these potbellied chickens have low cholesterol and triglyceride levels.

To see if SMAM-1 has a role in human obesity, Nikhil Dhurandar and colleagues tested fifty-two obese people and found that ten of them were infected with SMAM-1. These ten people were significantly heavier than the other obese people in the study. Like the chickens, people infected with SMAM-1 had unusually low cholesterol and triglyceride levels. The authors concluded:

> The presence of increased obesity, antibodies to SMAM-1, reduced levels of blood lipids, and viremia that produces a typical infection in chicken embryos suggests that SMAM-1, or a serologically similar human virus, may be involved in the cause of obesity in some humans.[12]

Adenovirus (type Ad-36). In a later study, Dr. Dhurandhar and colleagues showed that mice and chickens infected with adenovirus-36 (Ad-36) had twice as much fat on their bodies as uninfected animals.

What benefit does adenovirus-36 get from fattening up its host? A better home, apparently. Adenoviruses, like many other germs, can enter a latent phase in healthy people and then reemerge later if their hosts' immune systems are weakened.[13] Where do Ad-36 virions hide during these latent phases? In fat cells.[14]

Adenoviruses are often used in gene therapy to carry "designer genes" into the cells of patients with genetic disorders. A recent study conducted by NIH researchers suggests that adenoviruses used in gene therapy may stimulate the production of cortisol and other hormones.[15]

Borna disease virus (BDV). BDV causes encephalitis in horses and other animals. It has also been found in the brains of psychiatric patients. For years, it was thought that BDV did not infect many humans, but recent studies suggest that it may infect millions of more or less healthy people. Rats gain weight rapidly when infected with BDV,[16] but no one has studied BDV's effect on human weight.

Borrelia burgdorferi. *B. burgdorferi* is the bacterium that causes Lyme disease. It is transmitted to humans by ticks, and it cannot be spread directly from one human to another. Patients typically lose 5 to 10 pounds during the early, acute phase of the infection, then they begin to gain weight as the disease becomes chronic. It is not unusual for Lyme disease patients to gain 30 to 90 pounds, and some have gained 400 pounds. Ginger Savely, a nurse-practitioner who has treated hundreds of patients with tick-borne diseases, says that about 90 percent of her Lyme disease patients become overweight. People with Lyme disease have elevated cortisol levels and they almost never lose weight before their infections are cured. Lyme disease is no longer a rare malady—the U.S. Centers for Disease Control reported 23,000 new cases in 2002. You can learn more about *B. burgdorferi* and Lyme disease at www.lymediseaseassociation.org.

***Chlamydophila pneumoniae* (CPN).** The studies that have looked for links between CPN infection and weight focused on BMI measurements, not WHR or waist size. BMI measurements are not closely linked to cortisol levels, so we would not expect to find a strong link between CPN and BMI. Two studies did find weak links, however. H. Toplak and colleagues measured the BMIs of 119 patients and then tested them for CPN infections. They found that patients with higher BMIs were much more likely than lean ones to be infected with CPN.[17]

Swedish researchers tested 598 people for infections with CPN and *Helicobacter pylori*, the bacterium that causes ulcers. They found that 245 (41 percent) of the people tested were infected with both germs! The doubly-infected subjects had slightly higher BMIs than the other subjects.[18]

Helicobacter pylori. *H. pylori* is famous for causing stomach ulcers and cancer. Swedish researchers conducted a study to find out if *H. pylori* was an important risk factor for heart disease. They concluded that it wasn't. One of the unexpected findings was that men with *H. pylori* infections had higher WHRs than uninfected men.[19]

SUMMARY

Chapters 8 through 11 explained how hormones control blood sugar levels, fat storage, appetite, and our shape (apple or pear). We also saw that most of the disorders associated with obesity are caused by excesses or deficiencies of those same hormones.

The hormones that control our weight and appearance are controlled by our sex, age, the amount of stress we are under, and by common infections. We have very little direct, conscious control over our hormones, so we have very little direct, conscious control over our weight.

The next chapter explains what happens when we try to impose our will on our hormones by dieting.

REFERENCES

Epigraph: Quoted in *San Diego Union-Tribune,* Wed, October 18, 2000.

1. Kaye SA and Folsom AR. Is serum cortisol associated with body fat distribution in postmenopausal women? *Int J Obes* 1991 Jul;15(7):437–439.

2 Ljung T, Andersson B, Bengtsson BA, et al. Inhibition of cortisol secretion by dexamethasone in relation to body fat distribution: A dose-response study. *Obes Res* 1996 May;4(3):277–282.

3. Tuomilehto J, Marti B, Kartovaara L, et al. Body fat distribution, serum lipoproteins and blood pressure in middle-aged Finnish men and women. *Rev Epidemiol Sante Publique* 1990;38(5–6):507–515.

4. National Institutes of Health. 1998 May. NIH Publication No. 98-4098.

5. Lazarus R, Gore CJ, Booth M, et al. Effects of body composition and fat distribution on ventilatory function in adults. *Am J Clin Nutr* 1998 Jul;68(1):35–41.

6. National Institutes of Health. 1994. NIH Publication 94-3680.

7. Schaumberg DA, Glynn RJ, Christen WG, et al. Relations of body fat distribution and height with cataract in men. *Am J Clin Nutr* 2000 Dec;72(6):1495–1502.

8. National Institutes of Health. 1998 May. NIH Publication No. 98-4098.

9. Roome AJ, Walsh SJ, Cartter ML, et al. Hepatitis B vaccine responsiveness in Connecticut public safety personnel. *JAMA* 1993 Dec 22–29;270(24):2931–2934.

10. Birketvedt GS, Florholmen J, Sundsfjord J, et al. Behavioral and neuroendocrine characteristics of the night-eating syndrome. *JAMA* 1999 Aug 18;282(7): 657–663.

11. Chin K, Shimizu K, Nakamura T, et al. Changes in intra-abdominal visceral fat and serum leptin levels in patients with obstructive sleep apnea syndrome following nasal continuous positive airway pressure therapy. *Circulation* 1999 Aug 17;100(7):706–712.

12. Dhurandhar NV, Kulkarni PR, Ajinkya SM, et al. Association of adenovirus infection with human obesity. *Obes Res* 1997 Sep;5(5):464–469.

13. Isada CM, et al. *Infectious Diseases Handbook.* Cleveland, OH: Lexi-Comp Inc., p. 59.

14. Dhurandhar NV, Israel BA, Kolesar JM, et al. Increased adiposity in animals due to a human virus. *Int J Obes Relat Metab Disord* 2000 Aug;24(8):989–996.

15. Alesci S, Ramsey WJ, Bornstein SR, et al. Adenoviral vectors can impair adrenocortical steroidogenesis: Clinical implications for natural infections and gene therapy. *Proc Natl Acad Sci U S A* 2002 May 28;99(11):7484–7489.

16. Herden C, Herzog S, Richt JA, et al. Distribution of Borna disease virus in the brain of rats infected with an obesity-inducing virus strain. *Brain Pathol* 2000 Jan;10(1):39–48.

17. Toplak H, Wascher TC, Weber K, et al. Increased prevalence of serum IgA *Chlamydia* antibodies in obesity. *Acta Med Austriaca* 1995;22(1–2):23–24. [Article in German]

18. Ekesbo R, Nilsson PM, Lindholm LH, et al.. Combined seropositivity for *H. pylori* and *C. pneumoniae* is associated with age, obesity and social factors. *J Cardiovasc Risk* 2000 Jun;7(3):191–195.

19. Nilsson T, Lapidus L, Lindstedt G, et al. Relations between *Helicobacter pylori,* thyroid disease and cardiovascular risk factors in a 56-65-year-old population. *Scand J Prim Health Care* 2000 Jun;18(2):111–112.

20. Hill JO, Wyatt HR, Reed GW, et al. Obesity and the environment: Where do we go from here? *Science* 2003 Feb 7;299(5608):853–855.

12

Why Dieting Almost Never Works

In 2002, 64% of the U.S. population and 46% of the European Union's population were obese. By 2007, this figure is expected to reach 68% and 48%, respectively. Of these, only about 1%–5% will achieve permanent weight loss.

—DIET WATCHERS 2003, DATAMONITOR REPORT

Since you are reading a book called *The Potbelly Syndrome*, there's a good chance that you have tried a few diets. Did you think you had a fifty-fifty chance of losing weight and keeping it off? A one-in-five chance? If so, you were dreaming. Among independent researchers who have studied weight-loss programs, the optimists believe we have one chance in twenty of achieving permanent weight loss; the pessimists believe we have one chance in a hundred. Still, no matter how hopeless it is, people will continue to diet. This chapter explains why most of them will fail, and it discusses the dangers of succeeding.

WHY DO MOST DIETS FAIL?

Most diets fail because our bodies are exquisitely well designed to survive famines, and diets are voluntary famines. When we force our weight to drop below our appetite and fat-storage set points, we are fighting millions of years of evolution. An anonymous expert at the NIH describes it this way:

> Caloric restriction triggers a number of homeostatic endocrine responses including suppression of leptin, gonadotropins, sex steroids, thyroid hormones, insulin and insulin-like growth factors (IGFs) and elevation of growth hormone (GH) and cortisol. Some of these effects may be disadvantageous in terms of achieving loss of adipose [fat] tissue.[1]

In plainer English, this means that dieting suppresses the hormones that burn fat, and stimulates the hormones that store fat. Once again, it's really hard to fool Mother Nature.

Forty years after the United States declared war on fat, the National Heart, Lung, and Blood Institute (NHLBI) held a meeting to develop strategies for getting the public to lose weight. The meeting brought together experts from thirty-seven federal agencies and professional organizations. Considering that most of the speakers were dedicated anti-fat warriors, some very peculiar statements crept into their final report:

> • Stalonas and colleagues (1984) found evidence that patients regain even more weight than the initial weight lost. Literature on restrained eating by chronic dieters shows that dieting may result in increased weight. . . .
>
> • . . . chronic dieters have marked episodes of overeating that resemble binge eating . . . , and a subgroup of obese patients meet formal criteria for the binge eating disorder . . . , the development of which may be related to chronic dieting. . . . Excessive dieting associated with being obese may lead to binge eating, which in turn leads to increased obesity. . . .
>
> • Several researchers have documented the reduction in basal metabolic rate with calorie restriction. . . . The few patients who are able to maintain lower weights do so not by normalizing eating patterns but by continuing to restrict calories. . . .
>
> • The results of obesity treatment in adolescents have not been impressive. . . . Kramer and colleagues (1989) found that less than 3 percent of subjects were at or below posttreatment weight on all follow-up visits. . . . [2]

The experts quoted above were expressing what they had learned from years of study and analysis. Any overweight person learns the same things by the end of her second or third attempt to lose weight: Dieters undereat, then overeat; their weight is always going up or down, but mostly it goes up; there is never any end to dieting once started; and dieters are always hungry.

INVOLUNTARY DIETS

Calorie-restriction diets usually fail, but what happens to us when they succeed? Let's take a look at some extreme examples before moving on to the milder weight-loss schemes that you and I are encouraged to adopt.

Mother Nature performs experiments far too dreadful for any university laboratory. One experiment that She never tires of repeating is the testing of calorie-restriction diets. When children are chronically deprived of both protein and carbohydrates, they develop *marasmus*. Children with this condition are undersized and have very little fat on their bodies. They look like the survivors of death camps.

When children are deprived of protein, but still get some carbohydrates, they develop *kwashiorkor*. Children with kwashiorkor resemble the potbellied child in Figure 12.1. If permitted to eat all of the carbohydrates they want, these children will develop round "moon" faces and large deposits of fat under their skin. I have seen adult dieters develop this same look after losing a lot of weight and then regaining some of it. The weight they lost was from a combination of fat and muscle; the weight they regained was all from fat.

Whether these children have marasmus or kwashiorkor, they have high cortisol levels and low leptin levels.[3,4] Their thyroid levels are also low.[5] Their livers deteriorate.[6] They stop growing, and insulin resistance gradually converts the proteins in their muscles to glucose. The glucose created this way is enough to keep their brains alive, but not enough to allow their brains to develop. When these children are fed, their cortisol levels drop, leptin and thyroid levels rise, and they begin to grow again.[7] Their brains, however, will never recover completely.

As similar as the two diseases are, there are some differences. The children

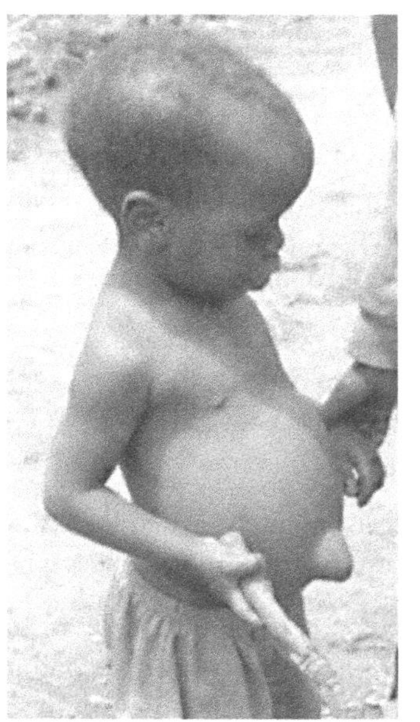

Figure 12.1. Child with Kwashiorkor

This child is suffering from an extreme protein deficiency, but has been getting some calories from carbohydrates. This condition is called *kwashiorkor.* (The protruding belly button is not a symptom of kwashiorkor.)

Children with kwashiorkor have cortisol levels roughly four times as high as healthy children do, and their potbellies are caused by deposits of visceral fat.

Children with kwashiorkor who get to eat a lot of carbohydrates may develop a cushingoid moonface and deposits of fat under their skin. This gives them a roly-poly look, so it is hard to appreciate that they are actually starving.

The photograph is from the cover of *ZIMBABWE,* August–October 2002. Physicians for Human Rights, Denmark.

with marasmus, who have been deprived of both protein and carbohydrates have higher cortisol levels and their muscles are consumed more rapidly than in kwashiorkor. The children with kwashiorkor, who have been able to eat some carbohydrates, have more damage to their livers.[8] The damage is in the form of *steatosis*, a condition associated with insulin resistance and diabetes.

Most of the research on marasmus and kwashiorkor focuses on children, but adults who are severely malnourished for long periods develop similar disorders.

DO ORDINARY DIETS KILL OR CRIPPLE US?

Do ordinary diets, the kinds touted in thousands of books and articles, cause symptoms of kwashiorkor and marasmus? Yes. Several of the experts at the NHLBI strategy meeting discussed the dangers of dieting:

> • Although studies show weight loss to be associated with improvements in blood pressure and blood cholesterol levels, weight loss also has been shown to be associated with higher mortality.
>
> • The adverse effects of very-low-calorie diets . . . can include ketosis; dehydration and electrolyte disturbances; elevated uric acid; body composition changes (losses of body water, bone mass, lean body mass); myocardial atrophy (which may result in congestive heart failure or sudden death); psychological changes (apathy); reduced physical activity; weight plateauing; rapid rebound weight gain upon refeeding; and a "rhythm method of girth control."
>
> • Yo-yo dieting. Repeated cycles of weight loss and weight gain may be associated with significant health risks. Hamm and colleagues (1989) have shown that the risk of death due to cardiovascular disease is twice as high for a gain-and-loss group compared with a weight-gain-only group.
>
> • . . . emphasis should be on [preventing obesity], not only because [reversing obesity] has such a dismal track record but also because of the questions that have been raised about the adverse health effects caused by weight loss and weight cycling.
>
> • Psychological problems commonly develop during dieting, and the risk of developing an eating disorder is particularly high during adolescence when dieting behavior is rampant.
>
> • Keys and colleagues (1950) found that a group of thirty-six psychologically normal males who were placed on about half their normal caloric

> intake—what is now considered a conservative treatment for obesity . . . developed significant emotional and behavioral changes during weight loss. . . .
>
> • Adolescent dieters experience increased incidence of anorexia nervosa, bulimia nervosa, and the binge eating disorder. . . . Both obese and lean dieters eat more when depressed than nondieters. . . [2]

If the statements quoted above sound incredible, keep in mind that they came from weight-loss experts at a conference sponsored by a U.S. government agency. Obesity may be dangerous, but weight loss is also dangerous. In the February 2002 issue of *Obesity Reviews*, there were two articles debating whether or not intentional weight loss increased death rates. The author of the "pro" article argued that intentional weight loss leads to more deaths in the long run.[9] The authors of the "con" article argued that intentional weight loss, on the whole, has no effect on death rates.[10] If losing weight has, at best, no effect, then why do our doctors want us to do it? I'll tell you at the end of this chapter.

CAN THINKING ABOUT FOOD MAKE US FAT?

You probably know from your own experience that diets seldom work, and even when they do, they leave you perpetually hungry and thinking about food. So this brings up an interesting question: Is thinking about the food you're not eating stressful enough to raise your cortisol levels? The answer seems to be yes.

Judy McLean, Susan Barr, and Jerilynne Prior performed an interesting study of sixty-two young, healthy, female college students. The subjects were tested to see whether they ate whatever they wanted, or whether they used conscious restraint to keep from eating some things. The subjects were divided into two groups—a low-restraint group and a high-restraint group. The two groups were similar in age, height, weight, BMI, waist size, hip size, and so on. The most significant difference between the two groups was that the women in the high-restraint group exercised more than the women in the low-restraint group.[11]

When the researchers measured the urinary cortisol levels of their subjects, they found that the women in the high-restraint group excreted 18 percent more cortisol than the subjects who ate whatever they wanted. An 18 percent difference in cortisol levels might not make much difference in a person's health in a year, but what will these high-restraint, high-cortisol women look like ten, twenty, or thirty years from now? I hope Dr. McLean will do follow-up studies to learn what happens to the women in each group.

A THOUGHT EXPERIMENT

Let's do a thought experiment where we combine what we know about insulin resistance, set points, cortisol, and dieting. Remember Clem from Chapter 9? Imagine that Clem still weighs 275 pounds. He feels fine, but he wants to lose weight so he can win the hand of the lovely Miss Meribelle. He has a morning cortisol level of 15 µg/dL, and his leptin level is 30 ng/ml (3 µg/dL).

Just for the purposes of this exercise, let's divide Clem's cortisol level by his leptin level. The result, 5, will be used as hunger- and fat-storage indices (this is not very scientific, but it is as scientific as most of the things we've been told about obesity). Remember, now, that leptin is produced by fat and your leptin level drops as your weight drops. After a year on his new regimen, Clem is a svelte 175 and looking pretty good, but his morning cortisol has climbed to 20 µg/dL and his leptin level has dropped to 10 ng/ml (1 µg/dL). This raises his hunger- and fat-storage indices fourfold to twenty.

All Clem thinks about is food. Since his sex hormones are suppressed by cortisol, he dreams of hamburgers instead of the lovely Miss Meribelle. His hair starts falling out. His muscles are so starved that they are breaking down their own proteins to provide amino acids to burn as fuel. His immune system is weakened, and he catches a new germ every week. He develops hypoxia (inability to get enough oxygen through his lungs) and he has life-threatening cardiac arrhythmias.[12,13]

Clem develops gallstones and winds up having his gallbladder removed.[14] Like a child with kwashiorkor, his liver begins to deteriorate.

Since his thyroid hormones are suppressed by cortisol, his skin becomes dry and flaky. His throat feels scratchy all of the time. The low thyroid also produces soft, flabby fat that is diffused over much of his body. He looks soft and feminine, except that his hair is falling out. His memory deteriorates. He can't sleep, and he becomes depressed and cranky. The lovely Miss Meribelle leaves him, taking his dog and his Elvis tapes.

If Clem stays on his diet, the excess cortisol will suck the calcium out of his bones, and he will develop osteopenia, osteoarthritis, osteoporosis, and osteonecrosis. His knees, hips, and back will hurt all of the time. His uric acid level will climb, and he will develop gout.

At some point, Clem will have a relapse and begin to stuff food in his mouth with both hands. Not all of the 12-step meetings on the planet will keep Clem from eating, and he will eat day and night until his leptin level is high enough to reduce his hunger to a manageable level. When Clem's weight stabilizes again, he will have less hair, less muscle, and more fat than he had before. He will look worse, feel worse, and have more medical problems.

Clem's experience was pretty bad, but it will get worse because his doctors and friends will talk him into doing it again!

The story of Clem is an exaggeration, of course, because most people abandon their diets or die before they develop all of Clem's complaints. Still, Clem's problems are common among dieters. If you haven't had an experience like Clem's, you probably know someone who has.

My brother and I both developed atrial fibrillations (rapid, irregular heartbeats) while we were in a weight-loss contest. This happened ten years ago and we are still plagued by fibrillations. My heart attack occurred a few years later while I was gloating over having lost twenty-seven pounds in two months.

EXERCISE IS BETTER THAN DIETING (BUT NOT MUCH)

What if Clem had tried an exercise program instead of a calorie-restriction program? Since moderate, enjoyable exercise can lower cortisol levels, Clem would have done a little better. He might have gained some muscle instead of losing it, and he might have retained his hair and his interest in Miss Meribelle. Clem wouldn't have lost enough weight to improve his love life, but it wouldn't matter much because he would have been too busy exercising to think about sex.

The following blurb from the NHLBI tells us what we can expect to achieve by exercising:

> Favorable metabolic effects were demonstrated in a study of six obese young men undergoing a 16-week walking program (Leon et al., 1979). The men exercised by walking on a treadmill for 90 minutes, five times a week, over 16 weeks. Overall, they decreased their body weight by 12.5 pounds. They also lost approximately 25 percent of their body fat, reducing their fat weight from 23 to 17 percent, while slightly increasing their lean body mass. Other favorable outcomes included reduced heart rate and blood pressure and improved glucose tolerance.[2]

These young men walked roughly the distance from Los Angeles to San Francisco. They burned an extra 88,000 calories, the equivalent of 25 pounds of fat, but they only lost 12.5 pounds. They walked 9.6 hours for every pound they lost, and they gained less than a half pound of muscle after 120 hours of exercise. Those are pretty small rewards for lot of dreary, repetitive, stressful work.

"Stressful" is an important word when discussing exercise. Your hippocampus is not very smart, but it is smart enough to figure out that something is wrong—stressful—if you are being forced to walk fast for long distances. It may not know whether you are chasing something or being chased, but it knows that you need stress hormones to speed you on your way, and one of those hormones is cortisol. Cortisol levels rise during any kind of exercise. If the exercise is moderate and enjoyable, cortisol drops below its normal level soon after we stop exercising. If the exercise is extreme or unpleasant, cortisol levels stay high for a long time.

If the young men in the treadmill experiment were sane, normal people, they must have dreaded every session. Their cortisol levels would have risen a couple of hours before they stepped on the treadmills, stayed high throughout each exercise period, and stayed high for hours after each session. The extra cortisol would have accelerated fat storage and inhibited muscle building.

From an evolutionary standpoint, exercise is only justified if it leads to food or sex, so the exercise you get from fishing, gardening, or dancing will probably do you a lot more good than the same amount of exercise on a treadmill. My guess is that the six young men in this experiment would have lost more weight, gained more muscle, and had more fun, if they had actually walked from Los Angeles to San Francisco.

Exercising to lose weight is such an unnatural act that it would be amazing if very many people succeeded at it.

WHAT ABOUT THOSE FORMERLY FAT PEOPLE ON TV?

We are bombarded with television commercials for magic drinks and sandwiches that are guaranteed to make us look like movie stars. These ads often feature spokespersons who claim to have lost weight and kept it off. Did they really? They probably did, but that doesn't mean we can.

Diets don't work very well, but people do lose weight occasionally, and sometimes they keep it off. I think some of the weight-loss success stories we hear come from people who have recovered from chronic infections. Remember the adenoviruses discussed in Chapter 11? They clearly make animals fat, and they appear to make people gain weight. Unpublished studies cited by the Associated Press, for example, found that 20 to 30 percent of overweight people, but only about 5 percent of the lean population, are infected with adenovirus-36.[15]

Researchers have found that animals with adenovirus-induced obesity return to their normal weights when the viral infection is healed. If this is also true of humans, then it may account for some of those cases in which obese people succeed in losing weight and keeping it off. The weight-loss industry may grab some of the ex-adenovirus patients and claim credit for their success in losing weight.

Several television celebrities have had gastric bypass operations, and they have lost weight and seem to be doing well. It's too soon to know what the long-term results of their expensive and dangerous operations will be. It is generally believed that gastric-bypass patients lose their appetites because their tiny stomachs get full quickly. Not so. The reason they lose their appetites is that their ghrelin levels drop sharply. Ghrelin, you may recall, is a hormone made in the stomach that stimulates appetite.

LOW-CARBOHYDRATE DIETS

Can you safely and permanently lose weight on "low-carb" diets? It's too soon to say. It appears that low-carb diets are effective ways to temporarily force your actual weight down below your fat-storage and appetite set point weights. In the end, your actual weight is likely to return to the highest one of those two set points.

Dr. Atkins, author of *Dr. Atkins' New Diet Revolution,* stated that low-carbohydrate diets do not raise cortisol levels.[16] I have not found any evidence to support or oppose his statement. My own efforts to lose weight on a low-carb diet were interrupted by my heart attack.

WILL LOSING WEIGHT IMPROVE YOUR HEALTH?

Losing weight would make some of us look and feel better, but there is little evidence that it will make us healthier.

There are strong statistical links between obesity and many other disorders. The medical establishment believes that obesity causes these other disorders, and based on that belief it has been urging us to lose weight for fifty years. When I tried to find studies showing that weight loss makes us healthier, I couldn't find a single one. Instead, I found statements like the following, all taken from NIH documents:

- . . . the benefits of long-term weight loss cannot yet be fully addressed because not enough individuals have sustained long-term weight loss.[2]

- Despite the compelling data for the benefits of short-term weight loss, there is little information regarding the health effects of long-term intentional weight loss in obese individuals.[17]

- To date there have been no randomized trials on the benefits of long-term weight loss because of the difficulty of achieving and maintaining weight loss.[18]

In other words, no one really knows whether losing weight will make us healthier, and we can't begin to study this question until someone devises a safe way to lose weight.

IS THERE ANY SAFE WAY TO LOSE WEIGHT?

There is no safe, effective, and proven way to lose weight. The ways that are effective are not safe, and the ways that are safe are ineffective or unproven.

The American Dietetic Association reported in 2002 that gastric (stomach) surgery was the most effective way to lose weight and keep it off, but only 50 to 80 percent of gastric surgery patients maintain their weight loss for more than five years.[19] Gastric surgery cannot be called safe. It kills from 1 to 2.5 percent of the patients who try it, and those who survive require lifelong medical attention to detect and treat complications.

Diet and exercise programs are not as effective as surgery, but they are probably safer. We don't know how safe these programs are, however, because none of them have ever been studied over a long period of time by independent investigators. The NIH is conducting a long-term study of a diet and exercise program called AHEAD, but the study will not be completed until 2012.[20]

I believe that most cases of abdominal obesity, and perhaps most cases of any kind of obesity, can be traced back to chronic infections. If this is correct, then the best way to fight obesity will be to fight chronic infections. This is, needless to say, an unproven theory.

SUMMARY

Our weight is controlled by hormones, not willpower, and obesity is caused in large part by an excess of the stress hormone cortisol. Chronic infections are an important form of stress, and hence a major cause of obesity.

Most of the disorders blamed on obesity are caused by infections or cortisol. Reducing weight safely and permanently is nearly impossible by any means available to us now, and there is very little evidence that losing weight will correct the health problems that accompany obesity. All of these points led me to ask, a few pages back, the following question: "If losing weight has, at best, no effect, then why do our doctors want us to do it?"

The answer is pretty simple. We would all like to blame our failures on some force beyond our control. For thousands of years, most people, including doctors, could blame their failures on evil spirits. In modern, industrialized countries, evil spirits are out of fashion, and doctors in these countries are now forced to blame their failures on fat.

Fat has been a wonderful substitute for evil spirits. When a patient fails to follow her doctor's advice and lose weight, the doctor can write off the patient with a clear conscience. A modern doctor cannot be blamed for the death of a fat patient any more than a witch doctor can be blamed for losing a battle with an evil spirit. Fat is the bad Ju Ju of the twenty-first century.

RECOMMENDED READING

Losing It: America's Obsession with Weight and the Industry That Feeds on It, by Laura Fraser (Plume, 1998).

Ms. Fraser skewers the diet gurus who exploit the hopes and fears of fat people.

REFERENCES

Epigraph: Datamonitor PLL. 2003 Nov. *Diet Watchers 2003.* Datamonitor Report No. DMCM0682.

Datamonitor PLC is an independent market research firm that is paid to provide businesses with accurate data.

1. National Institutes of Health. 2001. *The Effects of Dietary Carbohydrate and Fat on Hormone Regulators of Body Composition and Reproduction.* Clinical Study 01-CH-0183.

2. Strategy Development Workshop for Public Education on Weight and Obesity September 24–25, 1992 Summary Report. National Heart, Lung, and Blood Institute, National Institutes of Health, Bethesda, Maryland.

3. Soliman AT, ElZalabany MM, Salama M, et al. Serum leptin concentrations during severe protein-energy malnutrition: correlation with growth parameters and endocrine function. *Metabolism* 2000 Jul;49(7):819–25.

4. Van Der Westhuysen JM, Jones JJ, VanNiekerk CH, et al. Cortisol and growth hormone in kwashiorkor and marasmus. *S Afr Med J* 1975 Sep 20;49(40):1642–4.

5. Olusi SO, Orrell DH, Morris PM, et al. A study of endocrine function in protein-energy malnutrition. *Clin Chim Acta* 1977 Feb 1;74(3):261–9.

6. Guler A, Sapan N, and Salantur E. Effects of cortisol and growth hormone on the metabolism of liver and bone in children with malnutrition. *Turk J Pediatr* 1992 Jan-Mar;34(1):21–9.

7. Malozowski S, Muzzo S, Burrows R, et al. The hypothalamic-pituitary-adrenal axis in infantile malnutrition. *Clin Endocrinol* (Oxf) 1990 Apr;32(4):461–5.

8. Zeitlin M, Ghassemi H, and Mansour M. *Positive Deviance in Child Nutrition—with Emphasis on Psychosocial and Behavioural Aspects and Implications for Development.* United Nations University Press, 1990.

9. Sorensen TIA. Weight Loss Causes Increased Mortality: Pros. *Obesity Reviews* 2002 Feb; 4(1): 3–7.

10. Yang D et al. Weight Loss Causes Increased Mortality: Cons. *Obesity Reviews* 2002. Feb; 4(1): 9–16.

11. McLean JA, Barr SI, C Prior JC. Congnitive dietary restraint is associatied with higher uringary cortisol excretion in healthy premenopausal women. *Am J Clin Nutr* 2001;73:7–12.

12. Doekel RC Jr., Zwillich CW, Scoggin CH, et al. Clinical semi-starvation: Depression of hypoxic ventilatory response. *N Engl J Med* 1976 Aug 12;295(7): 358–61.

13. Van Itallie TB and Yang MU. Cardiac dysfunction in obese dieters: A potentially lethal complication of rapid, massive weight loss. *Am J Clin Nutr* 1984 May;39(5):695–702.

14. Liddle RA, Goldstein RB, and Saxton J. Gallstone formation during weight-reduction dieting. *Arch Intern Med* 1989 Aug;149(8):1750–3.

15. Associated Press, July 27, 2000.

16. Millennium Lecture Series Symposium on the Great Nutrition Debate, U.S. Department of Agriculture, February 24, 2000.

17. Study of Health Outcomes of Weight-Loss (SHOW), RFA DK-98-019, National Institute of Diabetes and Digestive and Kidney Diseases, November 18, 1998.

18. NIH Launches First Study to Examine Long-Term Effects of Weight Loss and Exercise in Type 2 Diabetes, News Release, National Institutes of Health, June 25, 2001.

19. Cummings S, Parham ES, and Strain GW. Position of the American Dietetic Association: Weight Management. *Journal of the American Dietetic Association* 2002 Aug;102(8) 1145–1155.

20. NIH Launches First Study to Examine Long-Term Effects of Weight Loss and Exercise in Type 2 Diabetes, News Release, National Institutes of Health, June 25, 2001.

13 Type 2 Diabetes

. . . a knowledge of sugar metabolism in animals will for long prove a difficult and laborious problem. Such knowledge must necessarily precede the elucidation of diabetes, but it must be remembered that diabetes is not a disease of carbohydrate metabolism alone, but is associated with marked changes in protein and fat metabolism as well.

—HUGH MACLEAN, M.D., D.SC., M.R.C.P, *GLYCOSURIA AND DIABETES*, 1922

Understanding diabetes is still a difficult and laborious task, but the task is easier if you begin by studying infections and cortisol, as we are doing in this book. Here is a brief description of diabetes from the National Institutes of Health:

> Although usually thought of in terms of . . . elevated glucose levels, diabetes is a complex metabolic disorder with abnormalities in carbohydrate, lipid, and protein metabolism. . . . Most diabetic patients die of cardiovascular disease (CVD), with CVD rates in diabetics two to four times those of the non-diabetic population.[1]

Roughly 16 million Americans have diabetes, and about one-third of them are unaware of it. Diabetes is the leading cause of adult blindness, lower-limb amputations, and end-stage renal (kidney) disease in the United States. More than 80 percent of all diabetics will die from some form of heart disease.[2]

TYPES OF DIABETES

Diabetes is a condition in which the body does not produce enough insulin to control glucose levels. Sometimes this occurs because the pancreas doesn't produce very much insulin, but more often it occurs because the body's cells resist the action of insulin (Chapter 8). There are four types of diabetes, and none of them are caused by obesity.

Type 1 diabetes. Type 1 diabetes usually strikes teenagers. It is caused by a defect in the pancreas that prevents it from producing enough insulin. Type 1 diabetics are usually lean, and weight loss—not obesity—is a problem. Their cortisol levels are a little high but they don't gain weight because their insulin levels are low. Type 1 diabetics require injections of insulin to control their glucose levels. This disease is often called insulin-dependent diabetes mellitus (IDDM).

Type 2 diabetes. This is the diabetes that tends to strike adults, and it is the focus of this chapter. Type 2 diabetics tend to be overweight, and like other overweight people, they have chronically elevated levels of cortisol and glucose. Their insulin levels tend to be high at first, then drop off as the pancreas becomes exhausted. Type 2 diabetics almost always suffer from insulin resistance (Chapter 8). This disease is often called non-insulin-dependent diabetes mellitus (NIDDM), and it accounts for about 95 percent of all cases of diabetes. Type 2 diabetes is the most severe form of potbelly syndrome.

Steroid diabetes. Cortisol-like medicines, commonly called *corticosteroids,* cause a form of diabetes that must be treated in the same manner as naturally occurring type 2 diabetes.[3]

Corticosteroids are often used to treat patients with asthma, arthritis, and other autoimmune problems, and these patients sometimes develop steroid diabetes. Corticosteroids are also used to prevent the immune system from rejecting transplanted organs, and transplant patients often develop steroid diabetes. A Scandinavian study, for example, found that 46 percent of the patients who received new kidneys eventually developed diabetes.[4] As with other diabetics, infections were a major cause of death for these patients.

One of the arguments we are making in this book is that a small excess of cortisol over a long time has the same effect as a large excess of cortisol over a shorter time. The same thing appears to be true of cortisol-like medicines. Researchers from Mexico City wanted to find out why some patients who were being treated with corticosteroids developed steroid diabetes while others did not. They studied fifty-four patients who were being treated with prednisone, half of whom had developed steroid diabetes. What they found was that the patients who developed steroid diabetes had received larger *cumulative* doses of prednisone than the patients who did not (27 grams versus 12 grams). The researchers concluded: "These findings suggest that high cumulated prednisone dose may induce DM [diabetes mellitus] regardless of another hereditary or personal predisposing factor."[5]

Gestational diabetes. Cortisol levels double during pregnancy, and pregnant women often experience symptoms of excess cortisol, including a form of diabetes. The babies of women with gestational diabetes are more likely to have problems such as macrosomia (large body size) and hypoglycemia (low blood sugar). Additionally, about half of the women who develop gestational diabetes will develop type 2 diabetes within twenty years of the pregnancy.[6]

TYPE 2 DIABETES AND THE DYSMETABOLIC SYNDROME X (DSX)

Richard Huemer, M.D., a noted author and lecturer, reviewed an early draft of this book, and he later asked me what I thought the difference was between type 2 diabetes and DSX. This turned out to be an important question, and looking for an answer led me to dig out much of the information summarized in Table 7.1, Disorders Associated with Potbelly Syndrome.

The answer to Dr. Huemer's question is that type 2 diabetes and DSX are the same disease, except that patients with diabetes have higher glucose levels. As the NIH puts it:

> Type 2 diabetes is the epitome of the [dys]metabolic syndrome.[7]

Dysmetabolic syndromes might well be called insulin-compensated diabetes, because the only difference between them and type 2 diabetes is the pancreas's ability to produce enough insulin to compensate for insulin resistance. Three Israeli researchers describe the difference between dysmetabolic syndromes and type 2 diabetes as follows:

> An insulin-resistant state—as the key phase of [dys]metabolic syndrome—constitutes the major risk factor for the development of diabetes mellitus. Hyperinsulinemia appears to be a compensatory mechanism that responds to increased levels of circulating glucose. . . . Fasting glucose is presumed to remain normal as long as insulin hypersecretion can compensate for insulin resistance. The fall in insulin secretion leading to hyperglycemia occurs as a late phenomenon and, in fact, separates the patients with [dys]metabolic syndrome from those with . . . overt diabetes.[8]

In simpler terms, type 2 diabetes is just DSX in a patient who can no longer produce enough insulin to control her glucose. Because of their higher glucose levels, type 2 diabetics often have more damage to their eyes, nerves, kidneys, and arteries than DSX patients.

Both diseases develop after years of chronic insulin resistance. In fact, insulin resistance is so central to DSX that it is sometimes called the *insulin resistance syndrome.*

INSULIN RESISTANCE AND DIABETES

In Chapter 8 we discussed the fact that cortisol's main job in the body is to keep glucose flowing to the brain under all circumstances, but we skipped a lot of details. Now that we are discussing diabetes, we need to take a closer look at how cortisol causes insulin resistance, DSX, and type 2 diabetes.

Figure 13.1 shows how insulin regulates glucose levels when we are not under stress (glucagon's counterregulatory role was omitted to keep the drawings simple). When glucose is a little low, insulin is also low, and only a small amount of glucose flows into our muscle, liver, and fat cells. As glucose and insulin levels rise, much more glucose flows into our muscle, liver, and fat cells.

Figure 13.2A shows what happens when cortisol levels rise a little and put us in a state of mild insulin resistance. Cortisol (not shown) makes our liver and muscle cells insulin resistant, which prevents them from getting very much glucose. The glucose level in our blood rises, and this raises our insulin level. The extra glucose and insulin partially overcome the insulin resistance so our liver and muscle cells get some glucose. Fat cells never become insulin resistant, so the combination of high glucose, high insulin, and high cortisol stuffs our fat cells with glucose. The fat cells turn much of that extra glucose into fat.

Brief spells of high cortisol and insulin resistance help us cope with life's ups and downs, and they do not harm us at all as long as they are interspersed with substantial periods of insulin sensitivity. When we become severely insulin resistant, we may not be able to produce enough insulin to force glucose into muscle and liver cells. Glucose continues to flow into fat cells, however, as shown in Figure 13.2B. This is type 2 diabetes. Muscle and liver cells are starved for glucose, but fat cells get too much.

Sometimes a patient's pancreas, after producing huge quantities of insulin for a long time, just gives up. Then, as shown in Figure 13.2C, glucose levels are extremely high, but there is not enough insulin to overcome the

A Low-Normal Glucose

Insulin enables liver, muscle, and fat cells to take up glucose from the bloodstream.

When glucose levels drop, insulin levels also drop, and liver, muscle, and fat cells cannot accept very much glucose. This prevents glucose levels from dropping too low, thus ensuring that brain cells (not shown) continue to receive an uninterrupted supply of glucose.

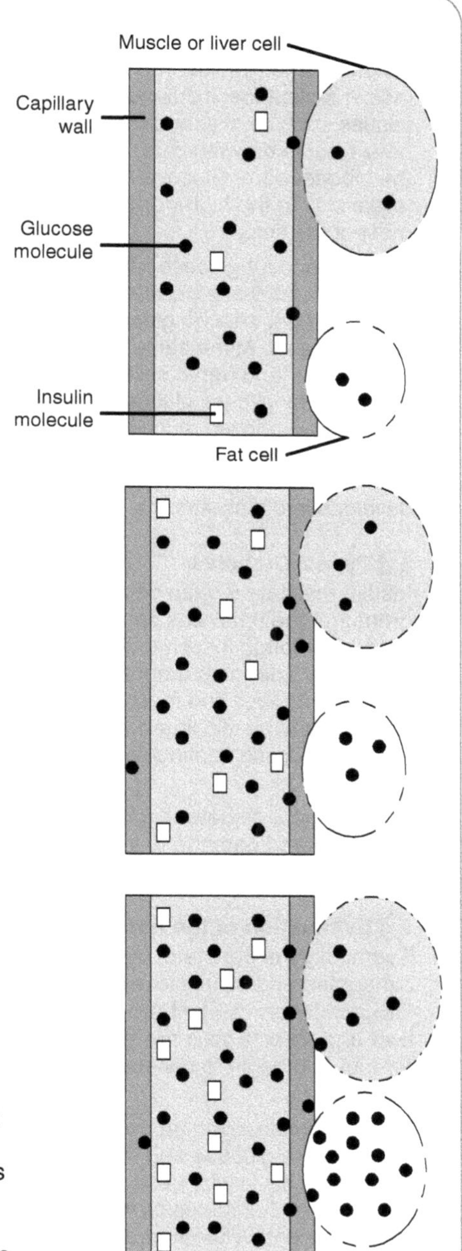

B Normal Glucose

When glucose and insulin levels are normal, then our liver, muscle, fat, and brain cells receive optimal amounts of glucose. They function properly, repair themselves easily, and they are not damaged by having too much or too little glucose.

C High-Normal Glucose

When glucose levels are a little high, the pancreas produces extra insulin to force glucose into the liver, muscle, and fat cells. This lowers glucose levels a little and protects brain cells and other insulin-independent cells from excess glucose.

Liver and muscle cells can only accept a limited amount of glucose, no matter how high our glucose and insulin levels become. Fat cells, however, convert glucose to fat, and they have a huge storage capacity on our waists and hips.

Figure 13.1. Normal Insulin/Glucose Behavior

A Insulin Resistance

When counterregulation develops into insulin resistance, insulin-dependent tissues such as liver and muscle cells have trouble drawing glucose out of the bloodstream. Glucose and insulin levels stay in the high-normal range most of the time.

Fat cells accept glucose readily, and turn it into fat, while muscle and liver cells can't get enough glucose to work properly. At the same time, kidney, eye, and nerve cells are being damaged by excess glucose. We feel "tired and rundown" much of the time, but sweets make us feel better briefly. This is potbelly syndrome before it develops into diabetes.

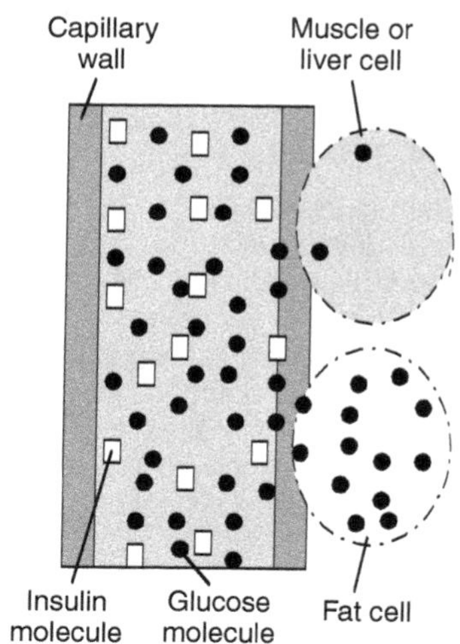

B Type 2 Diabetes

Insulin resistance often becomes so great that the pancreas can no longer produce enough insulin to force even marginally adequate amounts of glucose into liver and muscle cells. Glucose and insulin levels are very high, so glucose continues to move into fat cells.

This is type 2 diabetes, and there is widespread damage to tissues throughout the body.

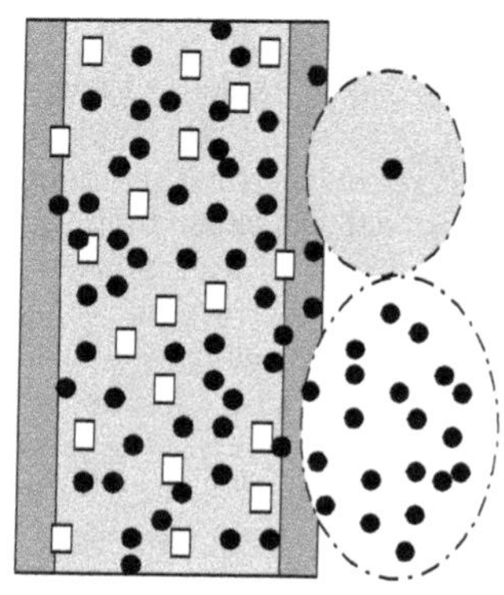

C Exhaustion of the Pancreas

Eventually the pancreas becomes exhausted and insulin levels drop. Glucose levels climb sharply, but liver and muscle cells are starved for fuel and begin to consume themselves.

Without insulin, even fat cells cannot accept more glucose and they begin to shrink. This is why people with severe type 2 diabetes often begin to lose weight. Without treatment, death follows quickly.

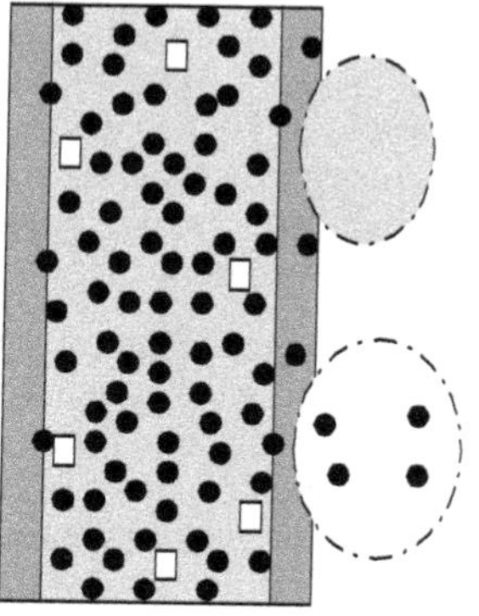

Figure 13.2. Insulin Resistance and Type 2 Diabetes

insulin resistance. Liver and muscle cells are damaged or killed by a lack of glucose despite the high levels of glucose in the blood. Without insulin, even fat cells cannot obtain glucose from the blood, so people with severe type 2 diabetes begin to lose weight.

Long-term insulin resistance damages most of the cells in the body by either exposing them to too much glucose (arteries, nerves, eyes, kidneys), or by depriving them of glucose (liver and muscles). Consequently, even when insulin resistance is corrected, it may take months or years for the body to recover completely.

INFECTIONS AND DIABETES

People with diabetes are more susceptible to infections than nondiabetics.[9] There is considerable evidence that the reverse is also true: Infections make people susceptible to diabetes. Several studies linking infections to type 2 diabetes are discussed below.

***Chlamydophila pneumoniae* (CPN).** There are no large studies of the relationship between CPN and diabetes, but there are hints that such research would be rewarding. For example, researchers from Sri Lanka found that coronary heart disease (CHD) patients with diabetes were more likely to be infected with CPN than were similar patients without diabetes. These researchers concluded, ". . . *C. pneumoniae* infection may be linked to CHD through its interaction with some of the known risk factors such as blood lipids, diabetes and smoking."[10]

C-reactive protein (CRP). CRP is a marker for inflammation and infection, and it is frequently found in overweight people, heart attack victims, and type 2 diabetics. Researchers from Mexico were interested in learning the relationship between CRP and glucose levels in diabetics. To do this, they measured the CRP and glucose levels of sixty-two type 2 diabetics and sixty-two control subjects. As expected, there was a close relationship between CRP and glucose levels. In fact, people with CRP levels above 10 mg/L were 7.4 times more likely to have hyperglycemia than people with lower levels.[11]

There was another important finding in this study. Half of the diabetics and half of the control subjects had been chosen because they were suffering from diarrhea or urinary tract infections (UTIs). The number of people in each subgroup who had CRP levels above 10 mg/L was as follows:

- Type 2 diabetics with diarrhea or UTIs: 30 of 31 (96.7 percent)
- Type 2 diabetics without diarrhea or known infections: 29 of 31 (93.5 percent)
- Nondiabetics with acute diarrhea or UTIs: 28 of 31 (90.3 percent)
- Nondiabetics without diarrhea or known infections: 0 of 31 (00.0 percent)

Note that type 2 diabetics *without any known infections* were slightly more likely to have high CRP levels than were nondiabetics suffering from serious infections. This suggests that diabetics have major infections that their doctors have missed.

Cytokines. J. C. Pickup and M. A. Crook, from Guy's Hospital in London, have suggested that type 2 diabetes is caused by a chronically activated immune system. Their theory, in a nutshell, is that marginally high levels of cytokines, especially IL-1, IL-6, and TNF-alpha, stimulate the production of acute phase proteins and cortisol. Over a long period of time, the excess cytokines, acute phase proteins, and cortisol produce all of the woes of type 2 diabetes, including heart disease.[12] Does this sound familiar? This is the same sequence of events that causes strokes, potbellies, high blood pressure, insulin resistance, RSX, and DSX.

Drs. Pickup and Crook do not explain why diabetics have high levels of cytokines, but I think the answer is obvious—infections.

Helicobacter pylori. *H. pylori* is a bacterium that causes ulcers and stomach cancer. Researchers from Italy found that women with diabetes were more than twice as likely as control subjects to be infected with *H. pylori*.[13] They also found that the *H. pylori* infections correlated with:

- Macroangiopathy (large blood vessel diseases)
- Neuropathy (nerve damage)
- Higher body-mass index
- Higher blood pressure
- Higher fasting glucose and HbA1c levels

H. pylori infections are very common, and they are relatively easy to treat. If you are diabetic and have any stomach problems, it would be worthwhile to have yourself tested for this germ.

Hepatitis C virus (HCV). HCV causes several diseases, including liver cancer. Researchers from Baltimore, Maryland, found that people over age thirty-nine with HCV infections were almost four times as likely to have type 2 diabetes as those without HCV infections.[14]

Human papilloma virus (HPV). This virus has been linked to type 2 diabetes. It is discussed in Chapter 3.

Immunoglobulin A (IgA). Immunoglobulins (antibodies) are produced by the immune system, and your IgA level indicates how heavily infected you are at any moment. If type 2 diabetes is caused by infections, then we would expect diabetics to have high IgA levels, and in fact they do. C. W. Gill and colleagues compared the IgA levels of five groups of people.[15] The groups, ranked from lowest IgA level to highest, were:

1. Normal controls
2. Hospitalized controls without bacterial infections
3. Hospitalized controls with bacterial infections
4. Type 2 diabetics without known infections
5. Type 2 diabetics with known infections

Note that type 2 diabetics without any known infections had higher levels of IgA than control subjects with known bacterial infections! This is additional evidence that type 2 diabetics have serious but hidden infections.

DIABETIC NERVE DISEASE (NEUROPATHY)

More than half of all diabetics have problems with their nervous systems. Autonomic neuropathy causes gut and urinary tract problems. Peripheral neuropathy can cause burning sensations and other pains. Neuropathy is best known, however, for cutting off feeling to the legs and feet. Since the patient feels no pain, infections often go unnoticed until they are so bad that the infected limb must be amputated. In the United States, diabetes-related diseases of the blood vessels and nerves account for more than 60,000 amputations every year.

Diabetics with the highest cortisol levels have the most trouble with neuropathy. Researchers from England studied three groups of people: twenty-five diabetics with neuropathy, nineteen diabetics without neuropathy, and eleven normal control subjects. They measured the subjects' cortisol levels every hour from 8:00 A.M. to 7:00 P.M. From this data, they calculated the cortisol exposure of everyone in the study. Here is what they found:[16]

1. Normal controls Cortisol = 2,694 nmol/L*
2. Diabetic patients without neuropathy Cortisol = 2,800 nmol/L
3. Diabetic patients with neuropathy Cortisol = 3,609 nmol/L

* nanomoles per liter

These findings suggest that cortisol causes or exacerbates neuropathy. The difference in cortisol levels between diabetic patients without neuropathy and the normal controls is not very large, but keep in mind that a small excess of cortisol over a long time will have large effects.

CATARACTS

People with type 2 diabetes often suffer from cataracts, and it has been assumed that they were caused by excess glucose. Excess cortisol may also contribute to the development of cataracts. Cortisol-like medicines are routinely used to cause cataracts in laboratory animals, and high cortisol levels are linked to cataracts in people with and without diabetes.[17, 18] Researchers from Scotland studied the eyes and blood of 1,000 cataract patients and 1,000 control subjects. The cataract patients had more evidence of diabetes, as expected. They also had more chronic infections, subclinical liver disease, and higher levels of cortisol. Taking cortisol-like medications increased their likelihood of having cataracts.[19]

SUMMARY

Corticosteroids, including cortisol and cortisol-like medicines, interfere with insulin's normal glucose-regulating function and produce insulin resistance. Insulin resistance increases as exposure to corticosteroids increases. A small amount of insulin resistance (counterregulation) is normal, but as insulin resistance becomes more severe, and longer lasting, it begins to damage cells throughout the body.

Insulin resistance combines with the other effects of corticosteroids, such as hypertension and abdominal obesity, to produce potbelly syndrome. The mildest form of potbelly syndrome is Reaven's syndrome X, which gradually develops into dysmetabolic syndrome X. The most severe form of potbelly syndrome is type 2 diabetes.

A good diet, pleasant exercises, and glucose-regulating drugs can relieve the symptoms of diabetes, and extend a patient's life, but they will have little long-term benefit if corticosteroid levels remain high.

REFERENCES

Epigraph: MacLean, Hugh. *Modern Methods in the Diagnosis and Treatment of Glycosuria and Diabetes.* London: Constable & Co. Ltd., 1922.

1. National Institutes of Health. 1999. *Prevention of Cardiovascular Disease in Diabetes Mellitus-Clinical Center Network.* RFP No. NIH-NHLBI-HC-99-16.

2. Diabetes Mellitus: Challenges and Opportunities, Final Report and Recommendations, Overview—Part 1, Summary of Scientific Accomplishments, Gaps, and Opportunities Identified at the Trans-NIH Symposium "Diabetes Mellitus: Challenges and Opportunities" September 4–5, 1997, Bethesda, Maryland.

Much of the "boiler plate" information on diabetes in this chapter was adapted from this and other NIH documents.

3. Corrigan EK. National Institutes of Health. 1998 Nov. *Nutrition and Lupus, Patient Information Sheet #9.* NIH Publication No. 90-3054.

4. Gunnarsson R, Lundgren G, Magnusson G, et al. Steroid diabetes—a sign of overtreatment with steroids in the renal graft recipient? *Scand J Urol Nephrol Suppl* 1980;54:135–138.

5. Raul Ariza-Andraca C, Barile-Fabris LA, Frati-Munari AC, et al. Risk factors for steroid diabetes in rheumatic patients. *Arch Med Res* 1998 Autumn; 29(3): 259–262.

6. National Institutes of Health. 1998 Aug. *Diabetes in African-Americans.* NIH Publication No. 98-3266.

7. National Institutes of Health National Heart, Lung, and Blood Institute. 2002 Sept. Third Report of the National Cholesterol Education Program (NCEP) Expert Panel on Detection, Evaluation, and Treatment of High Blood Cholesterol in Adults (Adult Treatment Panel III) Final Report. NIH Publication No. 02-5215.

8. Tenenbaum A, Fisman EZ, and Motro M. Metabolic syndrome and type 2 diabetes mellitus: Focus on peroxisome proliferator activated receptors (PPAR). *Cardiovasc Diabetol* 2003; 2(1):4. www.pubmedcentral.nih.gov/articlerender.fcgi?artid=153546.

9. National Diabetes Information Clearinghouse. 1999 Mar. *Diabetes Statistics in the United States.* NIH Publication No. 99-3926.

10. Mendis S, Arseculeratne YM, Withana N, et al. *Chlamydia pneumoniae* infection and its association with coronary heart disease and cardiovascular risk factors in a sample South Asian population. *Int J Cardiol* 2001 Jul;79(2–3):191–196.

11. Rodriguez-Moran M and Guerrero-Romero F. Increased levels of C-reactive protein in noncontrolled type II diabetic subjects. *J Diabetes Complications* 1999 Jul-Aug;13(4):211–215.

12. Pickup JC and Crook MA. Is type II diabetes mellitus a disease of the innate immune system? *Diabetologia* 1998 Oct;41(10):1241–1248.

13. Quadri R, Rossi C, Catalfamo E, et al. *Helicobacter pylori* infection in type 2 diabetic patients. *1: Nutr Metab Cardiovasc Dis* 2000 Oct;10(5):263–266.

14. Mehta SH, Brancati FL, Sulkowski MS, et al. Prevalence of type 2 diabetes mellitus among persons with hepatitis C virus infection in the United States. *Ann Intern Med* 2000 Oct 17;133(8):592–599.

15. Gill CW, Bush WS, Burleigh WM, et al. Elevation of IgA levels in the non-insulin-dependent (type II) diabetic patient. *Diabetes Care* 1981 Nov-Dec;4(6): 636–639.

16. Tsigos C, Young RJ, and White A. Diabetic neuropathy is associated with increased activity of the hypothalamic-pituitary-adrenal axis. *J Clin Endocrinol Metab* 1993 Mar;76(3):554–558.

17. Ogiso M, Hoshi M, and Nishigori H. Neutral and acidic glycosphingolipids in glucocorticoid-induced cataract in chick lens. *Exp Eye Res* 1999 Feb;68(2):229–236.

18. Watanabe H, Kosano H, and Nishigori H. Steroid-induced short term diabetes in chick embryo: Reversible effects of insulin on metabolic changes and cataract formation. *Invest Ophthalmol Vis Sci* 2000 Jun;41(7):1846–1852.

19. Donnelly CA, Seth J, Clayton RM, et al. Some blood plasma constituents correlate with human cataract. *Br J Ophthalmol* 1995 Nov;79(11):1036–1041.

14

Cushing's Syndrome

Cushing's syndrome leaves virtually no body tissue untouched. Left untreated, it results in progressive adiposity, myopathy, dermopathy (atrophy, stria, purpura, and hirsutism), psychopathy, glucose intolerance, hypercholesterolemia, hypertension, atherosclerosis, immunosuppression, and, ultimately, death.

—J. A. YANOVSKI AND G. B. CUTLER, JR., NATIONAL INSTITUTES OF HEALTH

Cushing's syndrome is so similar to potbelly syndrome that it requires a skilled physician to distinguish one from the other. Both disorders are caused by excess cortisol, but in Cushing's syndrome the excess cortisol is usually caused by tumors, not by stress and infections.

SYMPTOMS OF CUSHING'S SYNDROME

Drs. Yanovski and Cutler, quoted above, are two of the world's leading authorities on Cushing's syndrome. I hope they will forgive me for translating their words into plainer English:

> A large excess of cortisol damages almost every part of the body. Left untreated, it causes progressive weight gain, muscle weakness, skin problems (thin skin, stretch marks, patches of broken blood vessels, and inappropriate hair growth), mental problems, prediabetes, high cholesterol, high blood pressure, heart disease, weakened immunity, and, ultimately, death.

Dysmetabolic syndrome X (DSX), type 2 diabetes, and Cushing's syndrome are all very similar, and they are all caused by excess cortisol, but they differ greatly in the speed at which they develop. DSX, for example, may take thirty years to develop into a severe, life-threatening disease. CS can develop into a life-threatening disease in a year.

The most important symptoms of CS are discussed below. People with DSX or type 2 diabetes will have some of the following disorders, but people with CS will have most of them.

Hypercortisolism. Technically, *hypercortisolism* means any excess of cortisol, but usually the term is only used to indicate very high cortisol levels. Since people with Cushing's syndrome often have very high cortisol levels, the terms *hypercortisolism* and *Cushing's syndrome* are often used interchangeably in medical journal articles.

People with PBS rarely have morning plasma cortisol levels above 25 μg/dL, and it may take decades for their cortisol-related health problems to appear. People with Cushing's syndrome often have morning cortisol levels above 25 μg/dL, and their cortisol-related problems develop more rapidly—in months or years instead of decades.

Insulin resistance. People with Cushing's syndrome have insulin resistance ranging in severity from Reaven's syndrome X to type 2 diabetes. Insulin resistance is an intermediate cause of most of their other health problems.

Visceral obesity. Visceral obesity is abdominal obesity created by an excess of fat inside the abdominal muscles. Patients with CS accumulate large quantities of visceral fat even though their arms, legs, and buttocks may be thin.

Localized fat deposits. Localized fat deposits on the face, back, and belly are the classic markers of CS, but fat can be deposited in other places. Fat deposits in the eye sockets may cause the eyes to bulge out (exophthalmos). This may occur in up to half of all patients with Cushing's sydrome.[1] Fat deposits around the spinal cord (epidural lipomatosis) can cause patients excruciating back pain, which can be followed by paralysis.[2]

High blood sugar. People with high cortisol levels, including those with dysmetabolic syndrome X and Cushing's syndrome, usually have high glucose levels. Since glucose levels are checked much more frequently than cortisol levels, these people are often treated for diabetes, but they are almost never treated for hypercortisolism. Diabetes treatments, naturally, have little long-term value for people with hypercortisolism.

Infections. Since excess cortisol suppresses the immune system, patients with Cushing's syndrome are attacked by germs that don't bother most people. Wurzburger and colleagues described a CS patient with a cortisol-producing tumor on her right adrenal gland. She was chronically infected with three bacteria (*Proteus*, *Streptococcus*, and *Staphylococcus pyogenes*) and a yeast (*Candida*). Her infections could not be eradicated by medications, but cleared up after her right adrenal gland was removed and her cortisol level dropped.[3] CS patients not only have more infections than healthy people, but the infections hit them harder. Graham and Tucker studied twenty-three CS patients with various infections. Doctors were able to lower the cortisol levels of nine patients and all nine of them survived; the remaining fourteen died.[4]

Heart disease. Excess cortisol raises cholesterol levels and contributes to the development of atherosclerosis (Chapter 4). Most people with Cushing's syndrome will die from heart disease if their hypercortisolism is not corrected.

Diffuse obesity. Cortisol suppresses the thyroid hormones, so people with hypercortisolism sometimes have low thyroid levels. The resulting *hypothyroidism* will cause them to have fat that is diffused over many parts of their bodies.

Steroid psychosis. People with hypercortisolism tend to be unhappy and "neurotic." The earliest and most frequent psychiatric symptom of CS is depression, but anxiety, irritability, hostility, and thoughts of suicide are common. Mental aberrations are found in many long-term CS patients.

Stigmata. People with CS often develop clearly visible features called "stigmata." The stigmata include a moon-shaped face, the fat deposits described above, and purple stretch marks on their abdomens.

CAUSES OF CUSHING'S SYNDROME

At a Cushing's syndrome conference in 2003, several CS patients told me that doctors are unable to identify the cause of about half of all cases of CS. A doctor at the conference agreed with the patients. The known causes of CS are tumors, medications, and alcohol.

Tumor-induced Cushing's syndrome. In the United States, about 2,500 people are diagnosed with tumor-induced CS every year. About 85 percent of these cases are caused by tumors of the pituitary gland, but tumors of the adrenal glands, hypothalamus, lungs, or ovaries can also stimulate cortisol production.

It's not clear how many people are walking around with undiagnosed pituitary CS, but autopsy studies indicate that 25 percent of the people in the United States have small pituitary tumors.[5] A brief review of related studies suggests that about 5 percent of these tumors produce ACTH, a hormone that stimulates cortisol production.[6, 7, 8, 9, 10] If these figures are accurate, then there may be 3.5 million cases of tumor-induced hypercortisolism waiting to be diagnosed.

Iatrogenic (treatment-induced) Cushing's syndrome. Dr. David Orth, a researcher from Vanderbilt University and a member of the medical advisory board for the Cushing's Support and Research Foundation, estimates that 250,000 people develop CS every year as a result of taking cortisol-like medicines.[11] These medicines are used to treat asthma, arthritis, and other inflammatory diseases, and some of them can be purchased without prescriptions.

Symptoms can appear very quickly in iatrogenic CS. Doctors from the University of Virginia reported the case of a man who developed CS after a single injection of methylprednisolone. It took more than a year for his cushingoid features to disappear.[12] More typically, a patient doesn't develop CS stigmata until he has been treated with these medicines for months, or even years.[13]

Alcohol-induced pseudo-Cushing's syndrome. Drinking great quantities of alcohol for several years can produce a form of hypercortisolism called pseudo–Cushing's syndrome. Alcohol-induced pseudo–CS is identical to tumor-induced CS, except that it usually disappears three or four months after the patient stops drinking.

A CASE HISTORY

One Saturday morning, while strolling through a flea market, I saw an obese woman selling books from her wheelchair. She appeared to be about forty, but it was hard to tell her age. She had thin hair, a round face, large deposits of fat on her neck, and her belly flowed out over her knees. I hesitated for a long time, and then I asked her if her doctor had ever mentioned Cushing's syndrome to her.

She gave me a big smile and said, "Yes, I was diagnosed with Cushing's about ten years ago, when I was eighteen."

She went on to tell me that she had diabetes, cancer, and heart disease, and she had been hospitalized many times. Not once in her many trips to doctors' offices and hospitals had anyone mentioned Cushing's to her again. I didn't tell her how extraordinary it was that she was still alive, but I did tell her how to contact the Cushing's Support and Research Foundation. I also suggested that she call a medical malpractice lawyer.

Think about this for a minute. Imagine this young woman seeing dozens of doctors after having already been diagnosed with Cushing's syndrome. Imagine her being hospitalized for infections and heart attacks and cancer operations. Imagine medical students being brought to her bedside to examine her for ten years, and in all of that time, no one mentions Cushing's syndrome or hypercortisolism to her. Now here is the hard part—imagine your own chances of ever being diagnosed correctly if you have one of the milder forms of hypercortisolism.

WHAT TO DO IF YOU SUSPECT YOU HAVE HYPERCORTISOLISM

People are seldom diagnosed with Cushing's syndrome, or any other kind of hypercortisolism, before they develop the stigmata described above. Only a fortunate few will live that long, however, since most people with marginally high cortisol levels will die from heart disease, diabetes, or infection before they develop stigmata. If you suspect that you are suffering from hypercortisolism, raise hell until you are tested by someone competent to interpret the results of the tests. And don't wait ten years.

If you have tumor-induced hypercortisolism, there is not much in this book that can help you, but you have a good chance for a complete recovery after surgery.

If your hypercortisolism is caused by medications, work with your doctor to find a combination of medicines that will reduce your hypercortisolism as much as possible. Cortisol-like medicines are often used to treat inflammatory illnesses caused by infections; if you can cure the infections, you may be able to reduce the amount of medicine you need to take.

Do not stop taking cortisol-like medicines without the supervision of your doctor, since the withdrawal symptoms may include an extremely unpleasant death.

SUMMARY

Ironically, there may be an advantage to having extremely high cortisol levels. If your cortisol is middling-high, chances are you will die from heart disease, diabetes, or infection before anyone checks your cortisol level. If your cortisol is extremely high, you will develop the classic Cushing's "look," and there is a good chance your illness will be recognized and treated in time.

RECOMMENDED RESOURCES

For more information on Cushing's syndrome, contact:

Louise L. Pace
Cushing's Support and Research Foundation, Inc.
65 East India Row 22B
Boston, Massachusetts 02110
(617) 723-3824 or (617) 723-3674

Or

Cushing's Understanding, Support, and Help Organization (CUSH)
www.cush.org

Small, nonprofit support groups like CSRF and CUSH are always short of money—your donations will be put to good use.

REFERENCES

Epigraph: Yanovski JA and Cutler GB Jr. Glucocorticoid action and the clinical features of Cushing's syndrome. *Endocrinol Metab Clin North Am* 1994 Sep;23(3): 487–509.

1. Kelly W. Exophthalmos in Cushing's syndrome. *Clin endocrinol* 1996 Aug; 45(2):167-170.

2. Kaplan et al. Spinal epidural lipomatosis: A serious complication of iatrogenic Cushing's syndrome. *Neurology* 1989 Aug;39(8):1031–1034.

3. Wurzburger MI, Prelevic GM, Brkic SD, et al. Cushing's syndrome—transitory immune deficiency state? *Postgrad Med J* 1986 Jul;62(729):657–659.

4. Graham BS and Tucker WS Jr. Opportunistic infections in endogenous Cushing's syndrome. *Ann Intern Med* 1984 Sep;101(3):334–338.

5. National Institutes of Health. 1995 Feb. NIH Publication No. 95-3924.

6. Abd el-Hamid MW, Joplin GF, and Lewis PD. Incidentally found small pituitary adenomas may have no effect on fertility. *Acta Endocrinol* (Copenhagen) 1988 Mar;117(3):361–364.

7. Felix IA, Rodriguez Mendoza L, Guinto G, et al. 120 biopsies of pituitary adenomas studied by immunohistochemistry and electron microscopy. A clinicopathological correlation. [Article in Spanish] *Gac Med Mex* 1992 May-Jun;128(3): 289–295.

8. McComb DJ, Ryan N, Horvath E, et al. Subclinical adenomas of the human pituitary. New light on old problems. *Arch Pathol Lab Med* 1983 Sep;107(9): 488–491.

9. Sano T and Yamada S. Histologic and immunohistochemical study of clinically non-functioning pituitary adenomas: Special reference to gonadotropin-positive adenomas. *Pathol Int* 1994 Sep;44(9):697–703.

10. Tomita T and Gates E. Pituitary adenomas and granular cell tumors. Incidence, cell type, and location of tumor in 100 pituitary glands at autopsy. *Am J Clin Pathol* 1999 Jun;111(6):817–825.

11. Foreman, Judy, "Health Sense." *Boston Globe,* May 26, 1997.

12. Tuel SM, Meythaler JM, and Cross LL. Cushing's syndrome from epidural methylprednisolone. *Pain* 1990 Jan;40(1):81–84.

13. Wilson AM, Blumsohn A, Jung RT, et al. Asthma and Cushing's syndrome. *Chest* 2000 Feb;117(2):593–594.

15

Cortisol Production, Regulation, and Measurement

Cortisol performs vital tasks in the body. It helps maintain blood pressure and cardiovascular function, reduces the immune system's inflammatory response, balances the effects of insulin in breaking down sugar for energy, and regulates the metabolism of proteins, carbohydrates, and fats. One of cortisol's most important jobs is to help the body respond to stress.

—U.S. National Institutes of Health

Cortisol is produced by the adrenal glands, but its production is regulated by the brain. Consequently, our thoughts and habits play a role in determining our cortisol level at any instant. In this chapter, we will look at the way the brain and adrenal glands interact with each other. We will also look at how cortisol levels are measured and how those measurements are interpreted and misinterpreted. In later chapters, we will discuss the kinds of thoughts and habits that affect cortisol levels.

PRODUCING AND REGULATING CORTISOL

Cortisol is produced by the adrenal glands, and the amount produced is regulated by the hypothalamus and the pituitary gland. Collectively, these organs are known as the *HPA axis*, and its operation is described below.

Hypothalamus. The hypothalamus is a thimble-sized part of the brain that regulates body temperature, heart rate, sleep, hunger, thirst, rage, aggression, and cortisol levels. As shown in Figure 15.1, it receives stress signals from other parts of the brain and from the immune system. When the number of

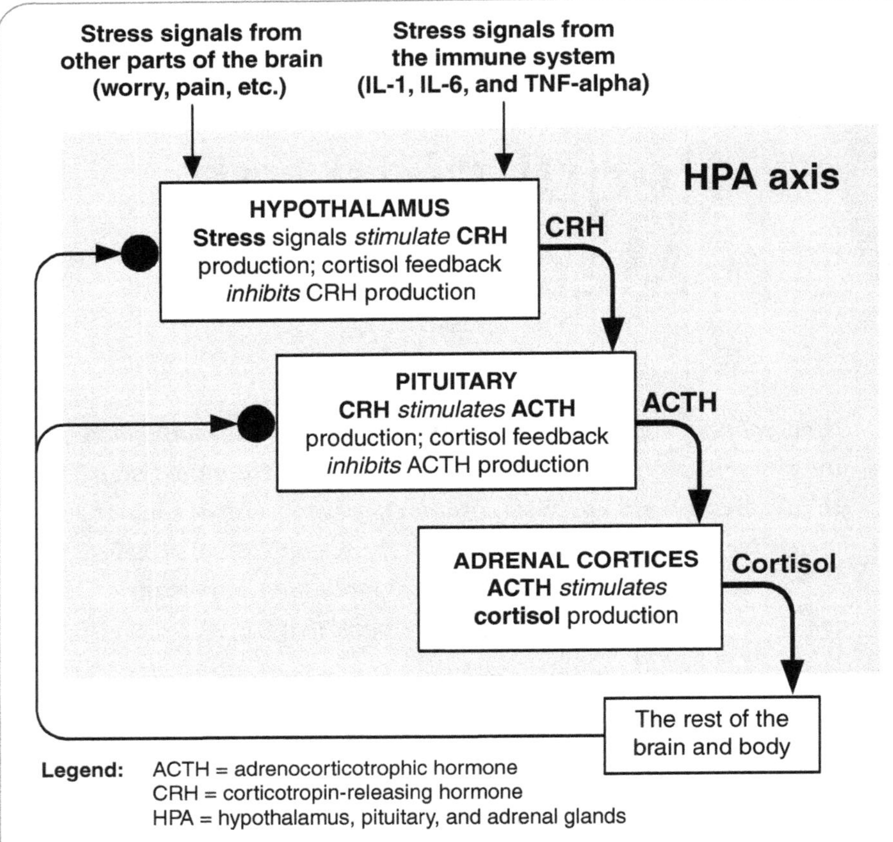

Figure 15.1. How Cortisol Is Produced and Regulated by the HPA Axis
Pulses of cortisol are produced by the adrenal cortex, but the number of pulses produced in a day is controlled by the hypothalamus. The bloodstream carries cortisol back to the hypothalamus and pituitary to form two negative feedback loops. These loops resist changes in cortisol levels.

As we get older, the hypothalamus appears to become less and less sensitive to negative feedback, and it triggers cortisol pulses more frequently than it should. This phenomenon may be a major cause of hypercortisolism in older people.

stress signals increases, the hypothalamus increases its production of corticotropin-releasing hormone (CRH).

As shown in Figure 15.2, the hypothalamus "weighs" the current cortisol level against the current stress level and decides whether to produce more, or less, cortisol. It is important to note that the amount of cortisol being produced when the HPA axis is balanced depends upon the amount of stress the hypothalamus senses. The HPA axis may balance with little stress and little cortisol (a good thing), or it may balance with a lot of stress and a lot of cortisol (a bad thing).

Many of the stressors that we experience come from our minds, not the world around us. For example, two women can be standing next to each other in a in a supermarket's quick checkout line. One woman is relaxed, imagining her next vacation, while the other is fuming and counting the items in the shopping carts ahead of her. The woman who is daydreaming is generating *antistressors* that will reduce her cortisol level, while the woman

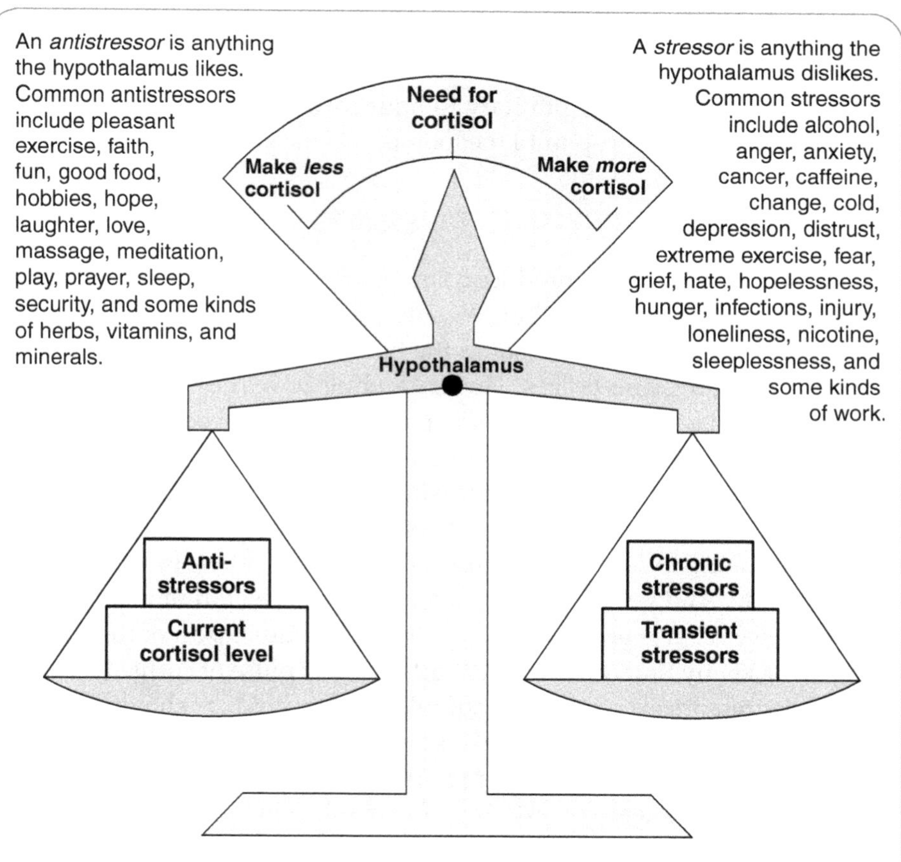

Figure 15.2. Stress-Cortisol Balance
The hypothalamus appears to compare all of our stressors with our anti-stressors and our current cortisol level. It then "decides" whether we need more, or less, cortisol.

counting grocery items is generating phony stressors that will raise her cortisol level. The hypothalamus is not smart enough to distinguish between real and phony stressors. That's a job for other parts of the brain.

Pituitary gland. CRH received from the hypothalamus stimulates the pituitary gland to produce another hormone called adrenocorticotropin (ACTH). ACTH is carried to the adrenal glands by the bloodstream.

Adrenal glands. The adrenal glands are located just above the kidneys. The inside layers (medullas) produce epinephrine and norepinephrine in response to nerve signals from the brain. The outside layers (cortices) produce cortisol in response to ACTH received from the pituitary.

The components of the HPA axis are arranged to form two negative feedback loops. Some of the cortisol produced by the adrenal cortices is fed back into the hypothalamus and pituitary to limit cortisol production. As cortisol rises, CRH and ACTH drop until the loop is "balanced" and stops changing.

BACKGROUND AND TRANSIENT STRESSORS

The adrenal cortices do not produce a smooth flow of cortisol. Under normal circumstances, they produce about twenty pulses of cortisol each day. After each pulse, the amount of cortisol in the blood rises quickly, then begins to fall until the next pulse occurs. Understanding how these pulses are produced can help us reduce the number of them that occur each day.

The things that annoy, frighten, or harm us can be divided, roughly, into background (long-term) and transient (short-term) stressors. Even the healthiest and happiest people have numerous background stressors pressing on them at all times, and transient stressors (stress spikes) occur frequently in everyone's life. And yet we do not get a pulse of cortisol from every stressor we experience. That is because the hypothalamus adds up all of the stressors acting on us at any time, and it only triggers a new pulse of cortisol when the sum of all stressors exceeds a cortisol-release threshold, as shown in Figure 15.3. When the cortisol-release threshold is exceeded, the hypothalamus releases a dollop of CRH, which triggers the release of a dollop of ACTH, which triggers the release of a dollop of cortisol. Some of the cortisol is carried back to the hypothalamus and pituitary, as shown in Figure 15.1, to provide negative feedback.

The cortisol-release threshold is regulated in part by the amount of cortisol in the blood, so the threshold rises after each pulse and then slowly drops

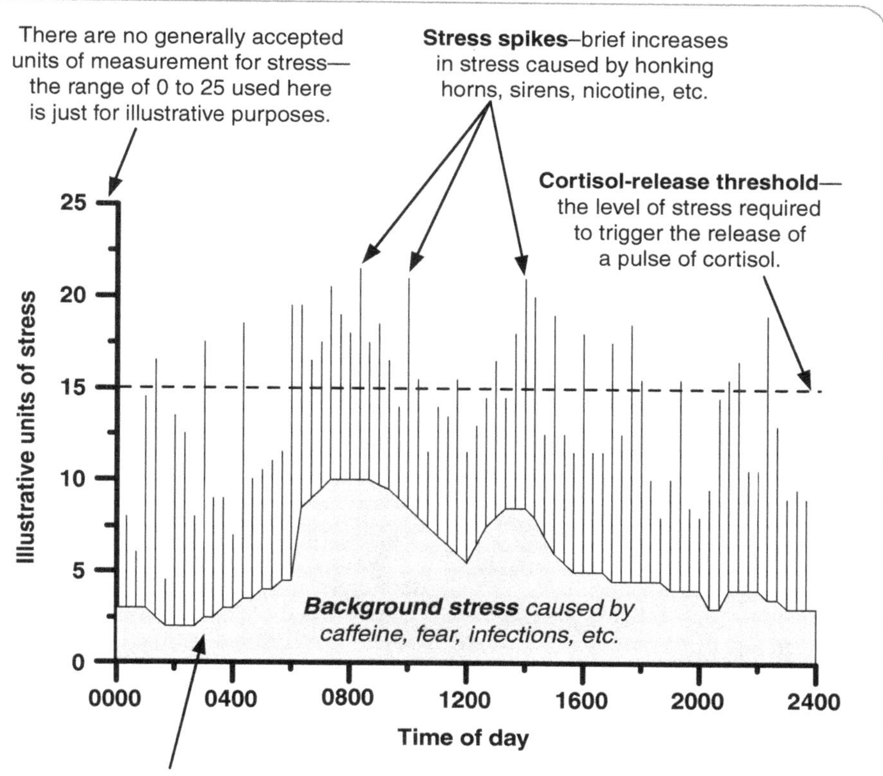

Figure 15.3. Stress "Spikes" Trigger Pulses of Cortisol

Our total stress burden at any moment is the sum of our background stress and transient "spikes" of stress. If we could plot our stress level on a graph, the spikes would appear to sit on top of our background stress, as shown above. Each spike that is high enough to cross the *cortisol-release threshold* triggers the release of a single pulse of cortisol.

Each pulse produces roughly 1 milligram of cortisol, regardless of the size of the triggering stress spike. Consequently, our cortisol levels are determined by the number, not the size, of the triggering stress spikes. In this illustration, thirty stress spikes cross the cortisol-release threshold.

as our cortisol level drops. When cortisol levels are high, it takes a lot of stress to trigger a pulse; when cortisol is low, it only takes a little stress to trigger a pulse. The constantly varying cortisol-release threshold provides negative feedback that tends to keep our cortisol levels stable.

The more often cortisol pulses occur, the higher our cortisol levels will be. In the example shown in Figure 15.3, the total stress exceeds the cortisol-release threshold thirty times. This would release roughly 30 milligrams of cortisol into our blood in one day. Thirty milligrams a day is pretty high, but it would not affect your health if you only produced that much cortisol for one or two days a week. If you produce that much every day for years, however, you will develop a potbelly and a number of potbelly-related problems.

If we can reorganize our life to reduce the level of our background stress, then fewer of the transient stressors will trigger the release of cortisol (Figure 15.4).

If we can reorganize our life a little more to reduce the number or size of our transient stressors, we can make a further reduction in the amount of cortisol produced each day (Figure 15.5).

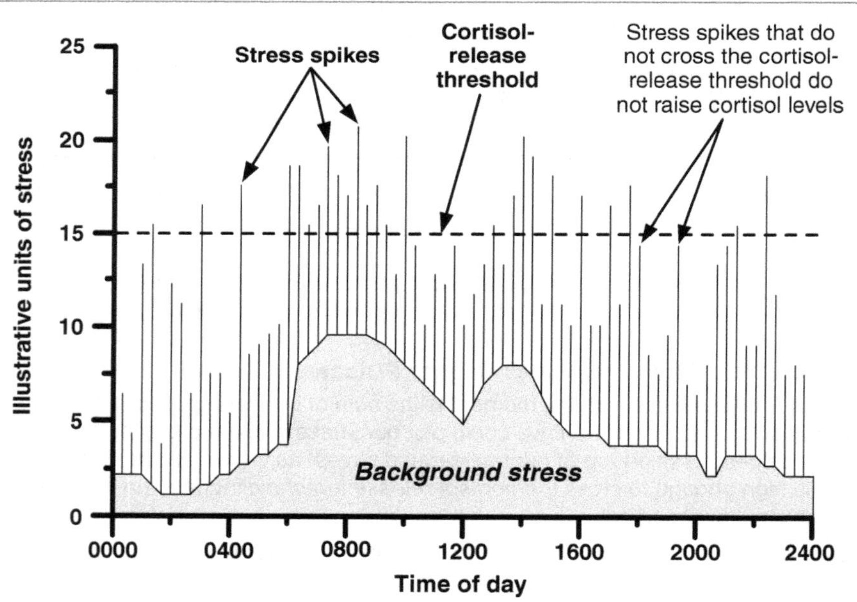

Figure 15.4. Reducing Background Stress Reduces the Number of Cortisol Pulses Released Each Day

Even a small reduction in background stress may greatly improve our health. In this example, lowering background stress one unit below the level shown on Figure 15.3 reduces the number of cortisol pulses from thirty to twenty-five. In real life, eliminating five cortisol pulses a day would result in a substantial reduction in our cortisol levels, with corresponding reductions in our weight and blood pressure.

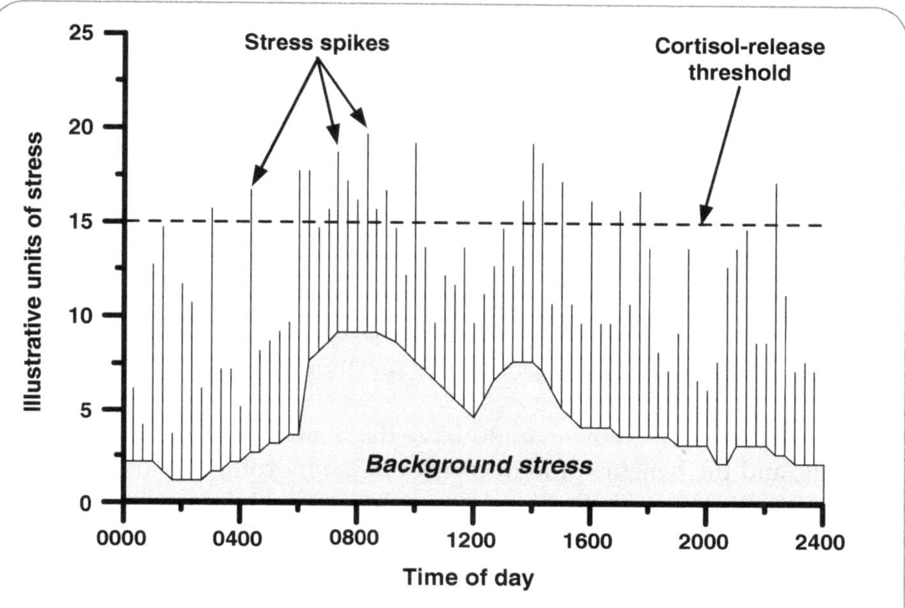

Figure 15.5. Reducing Stress Spike Size Reduces the Number of Cortisol Pulses Released Each Day

In this example, making each stress spike one unit smaller than the ones shown on Figures 15.3 and 15.4 reduces the number of cortisol pulses from twenty-five to twenty. Twenty pulses of cortisol a day is about average for healthy young people.

There are activities, such as meditation and pleasant exercise, that act as antistressors. They cancel stressors by some unknown mechanism. We can lower our cortisol levels by avoiding stressors and maximizing the number of antistressors we experience every day (Chapters 18 and 19). Is there any danger of making our lives so healthy, happy, and tranquil that our cortisol will be too low? I don't think so, but if you manage to do it, let me know your secret.

MEASURING CORTISOL LEVELS

Cortisol levels can be measured in blood, saliva, and urine. Tests to determine blood (plasma) cortisol levels are inexpensive, and they are available everywhere. Tests for cortisol in saliva are easy and inexpensive, but they are new and not widely used. Urine tests are more complicated and expensive, but they are also more useful.

Measuring cortisol is easy; interpreting the measurements is the tricky part. If you suspect that you have cortisol-related health problems, you should see an endocrinologist. At the same time, remember that most endocrinologists know very little about infections or the ability of infections to raise cortisol levels. Some of the factors that need to be considered when interpreting cortisol measurements are discussed below.

Diurnal cycles. In healthy people, cortisol levels are always changing. When you stand up, sit down, walk, talk, sleep, eat, or fast, you may be changing your cortisol levels. And even if you are doing nothing, there is a twenty-four-hour diurnal cycle with a peak in the morning and a dip at night (Figure 15.6).

The diurnal cycle allows you to have the benefits of low cortisol in the evenings, and the benefits of high cortisol in the mornings. In the evenings, when cortisol is low, your immune system is working hard to kill germs and your body is busy building and repairing cells. These activities intensify at nighttime. In the morning, the extra cortisol is stimulating and helps you start each new day with a burst of energy.

Flattened diurnal cycles. People with hypercortisolism tend to have flattened diurnal cycles, with evening levels higher than normal. Their morning cortisol levels may be normal, or even a little bit low, but their overall daily exposure to cortisol is still higher than it should be. Figure 15.7 illustrates how flattened diurnal cycles increase our overall exposure to cortisol.

Germs attack us around the clock, so infections tend to produce flattened diurnal cycles. AIDS patients, for example, do not have spectacularly high cortisol levels in the morning, but their diurnal cycles are flattened so that their daily exposure to cortisol is much higher than it would be in a healthy person.

People with flattened cortisol curves lose some of the anti-inflammatory benefits of high cortisol in the morning. They also lose the metabolic and immune benefits of low cortisol in the evening.

Morning and afternoon cortisol levels. The NIH's "reference" (normal) range for morning cortisol is 5 to 25 micrograms per deciliter (µg/dL). This range reflects the cortisol levels of normal people, not healthy people, so it is too wide. If your morning cortisol level is 25 mg/dL, you have a problem.

There can be large errors in measuring morning cortisol levels. The peak cortisol level usually occurs between 6:00 A.M. and 10:00 A.M. If your cortisol

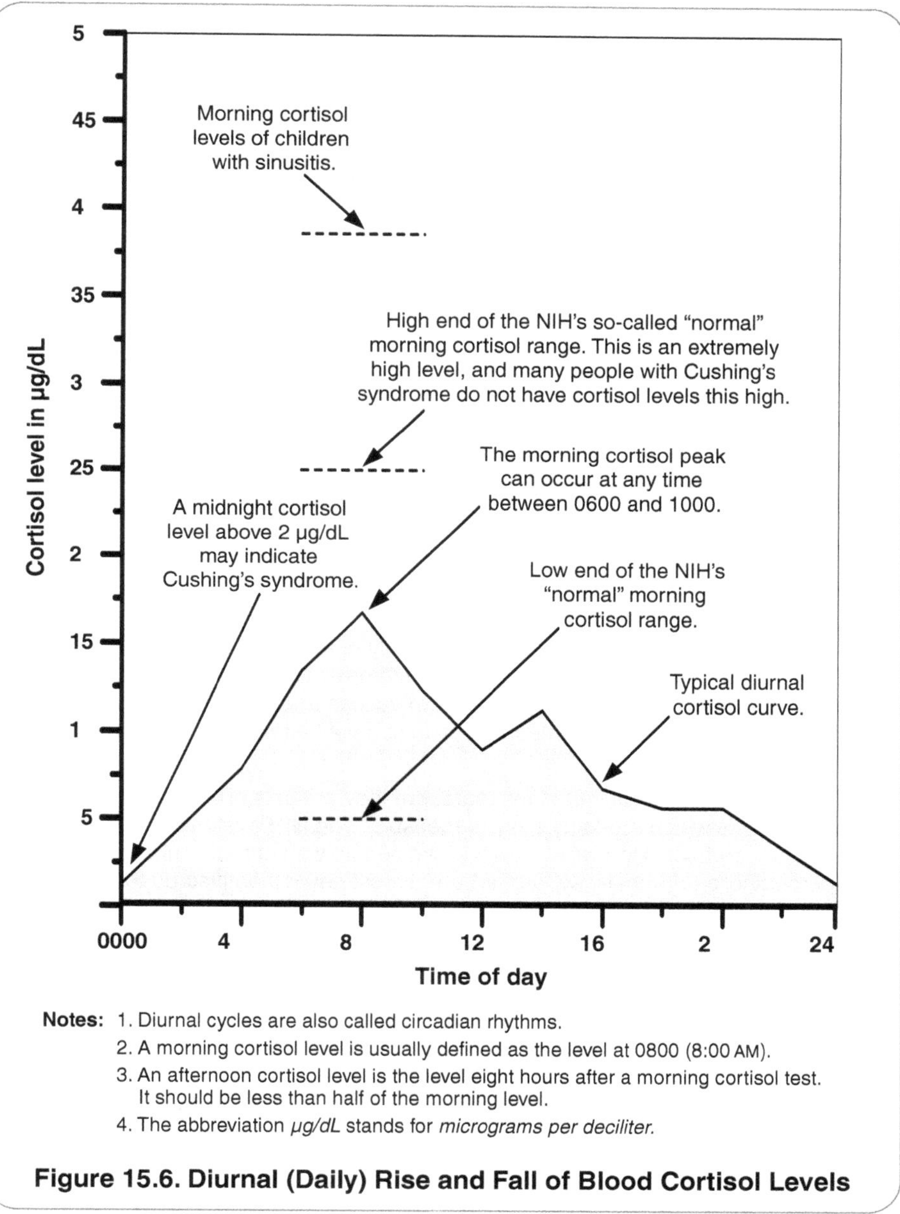

Notes: 1. Diurnal cycles are also called circadian rhythms.
2. A morning cortisol level is usually defined as the level at 0800 (8:00 AM).
3. An afternoon cortisol level is the level eight hours after a morning cortisol test. It should be less than half of the morning level.
4. The abbreviation *µg/dL* stands for *micrograms per deciliter.*

Figure 15.6. Diurnal (Daily) Rise and Fall of Blood Cortisol Levels

is checked only at 8:00 A.M., you could miss the peak by two hours. Morning cortisol tests would be more accurate if they were done at 7:00, 8:00, and 9:00 A.M., and the highest reading was used, but this is almost never done.

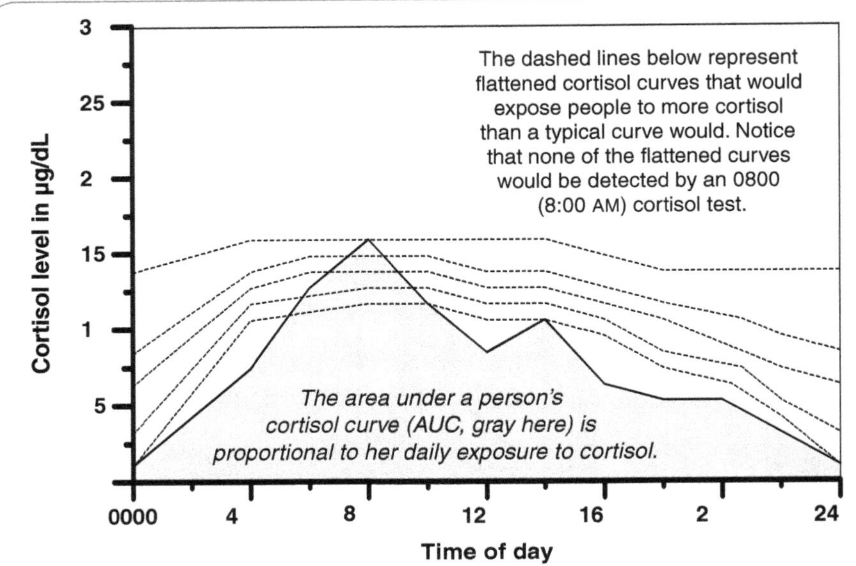

Figure 15.7. Flattened Diurnal Cortisol Curves

The damage done by excess cortisol is closely related to the area under the diurnal cortisol curve (AUC), and all of the flattened curves drawn above have larger AUCs than the typical curve does. Infections are stressful twenty-four hours a day, so people with infections tend to have flattened cortisol curves and large AUCs.

AUCs are extremely difficult to measure, but they are proportional to urinary cortisol levels which are fairly easy to measure. The NIH's reference range for urinary cortisol is too wide, however, so people with chronic subtle hypercortisolism (potbelly syndrome) are almost never identified on the basis of urinary cortisol measurements.

Comparing the results of morning and afternoon cortisol measurements would reveal all five of the flattened curves represented above, and a midnight cortisol test would reveal four of them.

Morning cortisol levels are not very useful, even when they are accurate, because they cannot detect the presence of flattened diurnal cycles. Doctors who understand this will have your cortisol levels measured in the morning and again in the afternoon. Your cortisol level at 4:00 P.M. should be less than half of the level it was at 8:00 A.M. Despite their many limitations, morning cortisol measurements remain important from a historical standpoint. Most of the older studies only measured morning cortisol levels, and we will have to rely on the information in those studies for years to come.

Figure 15.8 shows the morning cortisol levels associated with various infections and conditions. The scale goes up to 100 μg/dL, but levels above 25 μg/dL are unusual. People with cortisol levels above 100 μg/dL are in extreme danger from hypertension, catabolic destruction of muscles, heart attacks, strokes, fatal infections, and complications of diabetes.

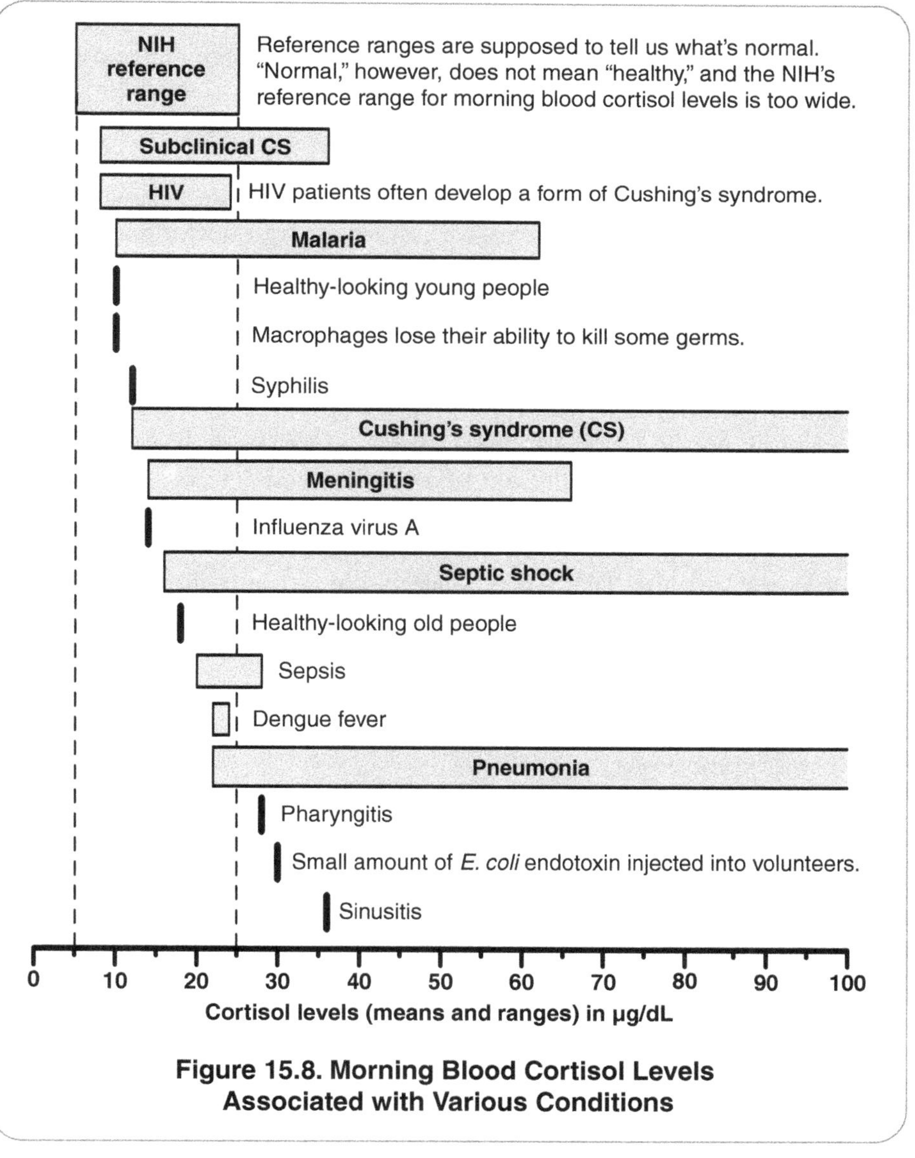

Figure 15.8. Morning Blood Cortisol Levels Associated with Various Conditions

Urinary cortisol levels. The purpose of a urinary cortisol test is to find out how much cortisol you produce during the course of a day. This is a valuable test, but it is an annoying one because you must collect all of your urine for a full day. A laboratory technician will measure the amount of cortisol in a sample of the urine, then she will calculate the total amount of cortisol you secreted during the twenty-four-hour period. Reference ranges for urinary cortisol, like the ones for morning cortisol, are too wide to be completely trustworthy. If your urinary cortisol level is within the reference range for the test you take, but it is near the upper limit, don't rule out hypercortisolism on the basis of that single test.

Dexamethasone (DEX) suppression test. Dexamethasone is one of the cortisol-like medicines we discussed earlier. If there is anything unusual about your morning, afternoon, or urinary cortisol levels, your doctor may give you a DEX test to see how well your HPA axis regulates your cortisol levels. You will be asked to take a DEX pill at midnight and provide a blood sample the next morning. If your HPA feedback loops are working properly, your cortisol level will be extremely low the next morning.

The standard DEX test uses 1 milligram of dexamethasone. This is a very large amount, and the test is so insensitive that almost everyone passes it. Tests using a fraction of a milligram are more likely to detect the subtle cortisol problems that cause potbelly syndrome.[1, 2, 3]

Midnight cortisol test. This test is relatively new, but it shows promise of being the single best way to determine whether you have hypercortisolim.[4,5,6] It is based on the fact that cortisol levels should be extremely low at midnight. If this simple test indicates that you do have hypercortisolism, then you may have to take many other tests to determine the extent and cause of your problems.

PARADOXICAL CORTISOL MEASUREMENTS

Research overwhelmingly supports the idea that cortisol causes potbellies and most of the illnesses associated with potbellies. Still, during my research for this book, I often found studies that seemed to show the opposite. As I studied cortisol, I kept asking myself: Why do equally skilled, talented, and truthful researchers get contrary results?

This question led to months of head scratching and rereading, and when I found the answer, it was so obvious that I wanted to kick myself for not figuring it out in an hour. Before I tell you the answer to this conundrum, let's take a close look at a study that appeared, at first glance, to find that high cortisol levels are good for you.

In 2000, Swedish researcher Roland Rosmond and two colleagues published a study showing that high morning cortisol levels were associated with extraordinarily good health. They studied 284 men, all of whom were fifty-one years old. Dr. Rosmond and his colleagues found that the men with the highest morning cortisol levels had the lowest BMIs and WHRs.

Fortunately, Dr. Rosmond and his colleagues measured each man's cortisol level seven times during the course of each day. After analyzing their data, they found that the men could be divided into two distinct groups, normal and abnormal cortisol secretors. The cortisol levels of the normal secretors were a little high in the morning, but they were very low in the evening.

The abnormal secretors had flattened diurnal cycles that were higher in the evenings, so they were exposed to more cortisol each day than the normal secretors were. Since it is the total exposure over time that determines how much damage cortisol does, it is not surprising that the negative effects of cortisol were found only in the abnormal secretors. The abnormal secretors were different from the normal secretors in every characteristic measured (Table 15.1).[7]

TABLE 15.1. NORMAL VERSUS ABNORMAL CORTISOL SECRETORS

Characteristic (✔ = yes, ✘ = no)	Normal cortisol secretors	Abnormal cortisol secretors
Cortisol is high in the morning	✔	✘
Cortisol is suppressed normally in DEX test	✔	✘
Cortisol level rises briskly after lunch	✔	✘
Flattened diurnal cortisol cycles	✘	✔
Blood pressure rises with cortisol	✘	✔
Body-mass index (obesity) rises with cortisol	✘	✔
Waist-hip ratio (potbelly) rises with cortisol	✘	✔
Blood pressure rises after eating	✘	✔
Heart rate rises after eating	✘	✔
Insulin rises after eating	✘	✔
Insulin/glucose ratio rises after eating	✘	✔
Triglycerides rise after eating	✘	✔

If you have a potbelly, you are probably an abnormal cortisol secretor. What would make you an abnormal secretor? Lots of things, but chronic stress and infections are near the top of the list.

A few pages back I posed the question: "How can equally skilled, talented, and truthful researchers get contrary results?" The answer turned out to be pretty simple. Researchers who only measure morning cortisol levels sometimes appear to find that high cortisol levels are good for you. Researchers who take multiple measurements of cortisol levels usually find that high cortisol levels are bad for you. The multiple measurements give a more accurate picture of our total exposure to cortisol, and they are the ones that we should trust the most. Measurements of urinary cortisol are in effect multiple measurements, and they nearly always indicate that high cortisol levels are bad for us.

CORTISOL SENSITIVITY AND CORTISOL LEVELS

There is one more reason why high cortisol levels may appear to be good for you, depending upon how a study is designed. This is a little more complicated than the flattened diurnal cycles, but it may be as important.

Cortisol molecules have no effect on us until they match up with cortisol receptors on our cells. When these match-ups occur, the cortisol molecules trigger chemical reactions in the cells, and these reactions change the behavior of the cells. During the chemical reactions, the cortisol is broken down into metabolites (breakdown products) that are carried out of our bodies in our urine.

If we are very sensitive to cortisol—that is, if we have a lot of cortisol receptors—we will break cortisol down so fast that our blood cortisol levels will actually drop. This will prompt the HPA axis to produce more cortisol, most of which will be quickly converted to more metabolites. People who are very sensitive to cortisol tend to have relatively low levels of cortisol in their blood and saliva, but high levels of cortisol and cortisol metabolites in their urine.

People with potbellies are extra sensitive to cortisol, and they metabolize it faster than thin people do. In a Brazilian study, researchers injected cortisol into obese patients. They found that the patients with the largest potbellies flushed the cortisol out of their bodies faster than patients with the smallest potbellies. In the words of the researchers:

> These findings indicate a more effective clearance capability for cortisol in

> patients with central obesity resulting in lowered cortisol plasma levels despite an increased cortisol secretion observed in this patient group. [emphasis added][8]

In a Swedish study, Dr. Mårin and some of his colleagues measured the amount of cortisol in the blood and urine of obese women. The women with the largest waists secreted the largest amounts of cortisol in their urine.[9] In another Swedish study, researchers found that obese men secreted the largest quantities of cortisol metabolites, but their *blood* cortisol levels were lower than those of thinner men.[10] These studies further illustrate how misleading a single morning cortisol measurement can be.

Why spend several pages talking about cortisol measurements? The reason is that a single morning cortisol measurement is nearly useless at best, and it can be quite misleading at worst. Nonetheless, most general practitioners, if you press them to measure your cortisol levels, will order a single measurement of your morning cortisol, and then they will tell you that it is within the NIH's ridiculously wide reference range. After that, they won't want to hear any more about cortisol, even if you weigh 285 pounds and have ten or fifteen clear symptoms of hypercortisolism.

FAT CELLS PRODUCE CORTISOL

It was discovered a few years ago that fat cells produce cortisol. This extra cortisol has profound effects on our metabolism, and at this time there is no known way of treating it.

Many of the body's cells, including kidney and colon cells, protect themselves from cortisol by converting it to a less active hormone called *cortisone.* Some liver cells and all fat cells reconvert cortisone back to cortisol.[11] The cortisone-to-cortisol conversion suggests that in addition to the infection-cortisol loop, some people may be stuck in a fat-cortisol loop that works as follows:

1. Cortisol helps produce fat.
2. Fat raises cortisol levels by converting cortisone to cortisol.
3. Repeat step one.

There is some recent evidence that fat cells only convert cortisone to cortisol when they are exposed to the inflammatory cytokines IL-1 and TNF-alpha.[12] Since infections produce both of these cytokines, people with infections may have higher levels of fat-derived cortisol.

SUMMARY

A pulse of cortisol is produced each time a person's total stress exceeds the cortisol-release threshold. This happens about twenty times a day in healthy, unstressed people, and more often in people who are stressed or who have infections.

We can reduce the number of cortisol pulses that occur each day by restructuring our lives and our thoughts to minimize stressors and maximize antistressors. There is a lot of evidence that this kind of restructuring can be done, but I haven't found any easy or fast way to do it.

Cortisol levels are constantly changing in healthy people. This fact makes measuring cortisol moderately difficult, and it makes interpretation of the measurements very difficult. Misinterpretations of cortisol measurements have prevented many doctors from seeing the strong connection between cortisol and potbelly syndrome. Dr. Mårin saw the connection many years ago, and in the next chapter, he discusses methods of diagnosing chronic subtle hypercortisolism, the malady that we have been calling *potbelly syndrome.*

RECOMMENDED READING

The Cortisol Connection, by Shawn Talbott and William Kraemer (Hunter House, 2002).

Drs. Talbott and Kraemer have backgrounds in sports medicine and nutrition, and this shapes their approach to reducing cortisol levels.

"The Endocrine System; An Overview," by Susanne Hiller-Sturmhöfel and Andrzej Bartke. *Alcohol Health & Research World.* Vol. 22, No. 3, 1998, pdf: 153.

This introduction to the endocrine system was prepared for health-care professionals, but it is so well written that anyone can read it. It is available for free from www.niaaa.nih.gov/publications/arh22-3/153.pdf.

REFERENCES

Epigraph: National Institutes of Health. 1996. NIH Publication No. 96-3007.

1. Barton C, March S, and Wittert GA. The low dose dexamethasone suppression test: Effect of time of administration and dose. *J Endocrinol Invest* 2002 Apr; 25(4):RC10-2.

2. Huizenga NA, Koper JW, de Lange P, Pols et al. Interperson variability but intraperson stability of baseline plasma cortisol concentrations, and its relation to feedback sensitivity of the hypothalamo-pituitary-adrenal axis to a low dose of

dexamethasone in elderly individuals. *J Clin Endocrinol Metab* 1998 Jan;83(1): 47–54.

3. Ljung T, Andersson B, Bengtsson BA, et al. Inhibition of cortisol secretion by dexamethasone in relation to body fat distribution: A dose-response study. *Obes Res* 1996 May;4(3):277–282.

4. Gorges R, Knappe G, Gerl H, et al. Diagnosis of Cushing's syndrome: re-evaluation of midnight plasma cortisol vs urinary free cortisol and low-dose dexamethasone suppression test in a large patient group. *J Endocrinol Invest.* 1999 Apr;22(4):241–9. PMID: 10342356 (PubMed—indexed for MEDLINE).

5. Newell-Price J, Trainer P, Perry L, et al. A single sleeping midnight cortisol has 100% sensitivity for the diagnosis of Cushing's syndrome. *Clin Endocrinol* (Oxf) 1995 Nov;43(5):545–50.

6. Raff H, Raff JL, Findling JW. Late-night salivary cortisol as a screening test for Cushing's syndrome. *J Clin Endocrinol Metab* 1998 Aug;83(8):2681–6.

7. Rosmond R, Holm G, and Bjorntorp P. Food-induced cortisol secretion in relation to anthropometric, metabolic and haemodynamic variables in men. *Int J Obes Relat Metab Disord* 2000 Apr;24(4):416–422.

8. Lottenberg SA, Giannella-Neto D, Derendorf H, et al. Effect of fat distribution on the pharmacokinetics of cortisol in obesity. *Int J Clin Pharmacol Ther* 1998 Sep;36(9):501–505.

9. Mårin P, Darin N, Amemiya T, et al. Cortisol secretion in relation to body fat distribution in obese premenopausal women. *Metabolism* 1992 Aug;41(8): 882–886.

10. Rask E, Olsson T, Soderberg S, et al. Tissue-specific dysregulation of cortisol metabolism in human obesity. *J Clin Endocrinol Metab* 2001 Mar;86(3):1418–1421.

11. Ibid.

12. Tomlinson JW, Moore J, Cooper MS, et al. Regulation of expression of 11{beta}-hydroxysteroid dehydrogenase type 1 in adipose tissue: Tissue-specific induction by cytokines. *Endocrinology* 2001 May;142(5):1982–1989.

16

Diagnosing Chronic Subtle Hypercortisolism

Researchers at the Centers for Disease Control and Prevention (CDC) estimated that as many as 47 million Americans may exhibit a cluster of medical conditions (a "metabolic syndrome") characterized by insulin resistance and the presence of obesity, abdominal fat, high blood sugar and triglycerides, high blood cholesterol, and high blood pressure.

—CDC NEWS RELEASE

Note to Readers Who Are Not Medical Professionals

Dr. Mårin wrote this chapter to help physicians diagnose chronic subtle hypercortisolism, the disorder that we have been calling *potbelly syndrome.* This material is more difficult to read than the rest of the book, so just skip this chapter if it is too technical.

Since the late 1980s, when Gerald Reaven introduced his mysterious-sounding Syndrome X, there has been a growing interest in *dysmetabolism,* the cluster of disorders that appears to begin with insulin resistance and then progress to type 2 diabetes and cardiovascular disease. Dozens of dysmetabolic syndromes have appeared in medical journals, newspapers, and books. Most of them share a core group of cardiovascular risk factors, including insulin resistance, obesity, dyslipidemia, and hypertension. There are about a dozen other factors, such as microalbuminuria and hepatic steatosis, which appear in some versions but not in others.

No single description of the dysmetabolic syndrome has risen to dominate the others because even the best of the currently popular versions have three major difficulties:

1. They cannot point to a single, central disorder that can account for all of the others, though insulin resistance comes close. Insulin resistance is so important that some experts refer to their versions of dysmetabolic syndromes as *insulin resistance syndromes.*
2. None of the currently popular versions of the dysmetabolic syndrome can explain why tens of millions of people are insulin resistant.
3. They do not lead to treatments of the syndrome itself—physicians must still diagnose and treat each factor independently of the others. Treating one factor will typically have little effect on the others, and it may in fact have a detrimental effect on them.

In this book, we are presenting yet another dysmetabolic syndrome which we are calling *chronic subtle hypercortisolism*, or more simply, *potbelly syndrome* (PBS). Chronic, subtle hypercortisolism overcomes all of the difficulties listed above. In short:

1. In chronic subtle hypercortisolism, the single, central factor that accounts for all of the others is *marginally supraoptimal glucocorticoid activity*, often called *subtle hypercortisolism.* The most important glucocorticoid is cortisol.
2. A normal part of cortisol's counterregulatory function is to create temporary states of insulin resistance. Chronic subtle hypercortisolism results in chronic insulin resistance, and tens of millions of people have both conditions. (Other people, perhaps tens of millions of them, have subtle hypocortisolism, but this book does not deal with their problems.)
3. Reducing glucocorticoid activity, whether by stress reduction, medication, or surgery, reliably reduces insulin resistance, visceral fat, blood sugar, triglycerides, cholesterol, and blood pressure.

Before discussing chronic subtle hypercortisolism in more detail, I'd like to digress briefly and review the development of the dysmetabolic syndrome concept.

BACKGROUND

The dysmetabolic syndrome concept has been evolving since the 1920s. In

1921, the frequently misunderstood psychiatrist Ernst Kretschmer published a paper linking certain body types to specific personality characteristics. Kretschmer published detailed circumference measurements, and from these it is clear that people with his *pyknic* body type had potbellies. Kretschmer found an association between the pyknic body type and mental depressive disorder. We know now, of course, that potbellies and depression are both closely linked to cortisol hyperactivity.[1]

A year later Felix Gaisböck described a syndrome in which hypertension and obesity were associated with psychological stress, smoking and alcohol excess in hard-driving middle-aged men. Cortisol had not been discovered yet, but in his article Gaisböck explained that the best way of preventing or treating the syndrome was to reduce mental stress. Reducing stress, of course, would have reduced cortisol levels![2]

In 1947, Jean Vague published data supporting an association between abdominal obesity and cortisol.[3] Very importantly, Vague was the first to measure cortisol metabolites excreted in urine. Cortisol levels are poor indicators of cortisol activity, but urinary levels are more reliable than plasma levels. Vague's findings were confirmed by Marcin Krotkiewski and colleagues in 1966.[4] In 1972, Herberg and colleagues described a "metabolic syndrome of obesity" consisting of five statistically associated components:

- Obesity
- Diabetes
- Elevated blood lipids
- Hyperuricemia
- Hepatic steatosis (unfortunately, this feature has been omitted from more recent dysmetabolic syndromes)[5]

There was little interest in the work of Kretschmer, Gaisböck, Vague, and Herberg until Gerald Reaven introduced Syndrome X in 1988.[6] After that, interest grew rapidly as the close association of dysmetabolic syndromes with type 2 diabetes and cardiovascular diseases became known. In 1998 the World Health Organization (WHO) presented a [dys]metabolic syndrome that was described as "a working definition to be improved upon in due course." Here is the WHO's definition:

- Glucose intolerance, impaired glucose tolerance (IGT), or diabetes mellitus and/or insulin resistance together with two or more of the other components listed below.

- Impaired glucose regulation or diabetes
- Insulin resistance (under hyperinsulinemic, euglycemic conditions, glucose uptake below lowest quartile for background population under investigation)
- Raised arterial pressure ≥ 140/90 mm Hg
- Raised plasma triglycerides (≥ 1.7 mmol l^{-1}; 150 mg/dL^{-1}) and/or low HDL-cholesterol (< 0.9 mmol l^{-1}, 35 mg dL^{-1} for men; < 1.0 mmol l^{-1}, 39 mg/dL^{-1} for women)
- Central obesity
  - Males: waist/hip ratio (WHR) > 0.90
  - Females: WHR > 0.85)
  - Either sex: body-mass index (BMI) > 30 kg m^{-2}
- Microalbuminuria (urinary albumin excretion rate ≥ 20 μg min^{-1} or albumin:creatinine ratio ≥ 30 mg g^{-1})[7]

Somewhat confusingly, the terms "impaired glucose tolerance," "diabetes," and "insulin resistance" appear in multiple places, so this working definition still needs a little work. Still, it is a sensible description of the syndrome. Four noteworthy features of the WHO definition are:

- Microalbuminuria has been added.
- WHR, which reflects central obesity, can be used instead of BMI.
- LDL cholesterol is not considered important enough to be included.
- Hepatic steatosis was not included.

In 2001, the U.S. National Institutes of Health (NIH) published a very simple definition of the syndrome.[8] According to this definition, the dysmetabolic syndrome can be identified by the presence of any three of the five risk factors listed in Table 16.1.

Interestingly, there is a little-known syndrome that shares the main features of the WHO and NIH dysmetabolic syndromes, from insulin resistance through hypertension. This syndrome, which is called subclinical Cushing's syndrome (SCCS), was discovered as a result of advances in ultrasound and computed tomography that revealed small pituitary and adrenal tumors in patients that lacked the usual stigmata associated with Cushing's syndrome. SCCS is indisputably caused by slightly elevated cortisol levels, and its

TABLE 16.1. CRITERIA FOR DIAGNOSING THE NIH'S DYSMETABOLIC SYNDROME

Risk Factor	Defining Level	
	Men	**Women**
Waist circumference	> 102 cm (>40 in)	>88 cm (>35 in)
Triglycerides	≥ 150 mg/dL	≥ 150 mg/dL
HDL cholesterol	< 40 mg/dL	< 50 mg/dL
Blood pressure	≥ 130/≥ 85 mm Hg	≥ 130/≥ 85 mm Hg
Fasting glucose	≥ 110 mg/dL	≥ 110 mg/dL

Note that obesity is defined by waist circumference instead of WHR or BMI.

symptoms disappear when cortisol levels are lowered. (See Chapter 7 for more details.)

Research done during the last eighty years strongly supports an association between subtle hypercortisolism and the common clinical features of dysmetabolic syndromes.[9,10,11,12] The evidence is not, however, so clear-cut, conclusive, and reproducible that everyone believes it. Some very capable researchers disagree with the conclusions presented here.[13,14]

The conflicting results of research in this field are due to differences in patient selection, study design, and, most importantly, differences in the methods used to evaluate cortisol secretion (basal, stimulated, inhibited, saliva, serum, urinary, etc.). When researchers measure urinary cortisol levels, or look at disturbances of the diurnal cycle of cortisol secretion, they tend to find links to the dysmetabolic syndrome. On the other hand, when researchers focus on simple measurements of cortisol in blood or saliva, they often fail to find such links.

Considering this background, it is not surprising that only a handful of physicians are aware of the disorders associated with small, long-term excesses of cortisol.

DISORDERS ASSOCIATED WITH HYPERCORTISOLISM

Each of the dysmetabolic syndromes discussed in this chapter is associated with a large number of disorders, and in each case someone has selected a subset of these disorders and used them as the criteria for determining the presence of their particular syndrome. Each set of criteria is a little different from the others, but they are all the same in one respect—they are all subsets of the disorders associated with hypercortisolism, as shown in Table 16.2.

TABLE 16.2. DISORDERS LINKED TO SEVERAL DYSMETABOLIC SYNDROMES

Disorder	Pre-Reaven	Reaven 1988	SCCS 1990s	WHO 1998	NIH 2001	PBS 2005
DISORDERS CLOSELY LINKED TO EXCESS CORTISOL ACTIVITY						
Hypertension	■	■	■	■	■	■
Dyslipidemia	■	■	■	■	■	■
Low HDL cholesterol			■	■	■	■
Central obesity	■			■	■	■
Elevated fasting glucose		■			■	■
Type 2 diabetes	■	■	■	■		■
Impaired glucose regulation		■	■	■		■
Insulin resistance		■		■		■
Hepatic steatosis	■					■
Hyperinsulinemia		■				■
High LDL cholesterol			■			
Depression	■					
DISORDERS LOOSELY LINKED TO EXCESS CORTISOL ACTIVITY						
Microalbuminuria				■		■
Diffuse obesity	■		■	■		
Hyperuricemia	■					

In addition to the disorders listed in Table 16.2, people diagnosed with a dysmetabolic syndrome are likely to have some combination of the disorders listed in Table 16.3. The disorders listed in Table 16.2 are present in most stages of hypercortisolism, but some of the disorders listed in Table 16.3 are found only in cases of severe hypercortisolism.

For a detailed review of the research linking obesity, diabetes, hypertension, and heart disease to chronic subtle hypercortisolism, see the earlier chapters of this book.

MARGINALLY SUPRAOPTIMAL GLUCOCORTICOID ACTIVITY

The inelegant expression *marginally supraoptimal glucocorticoid activity* was chosen to describe the cause of chronic subtle hypercortisolism/potbelly syndrome as succinctly and accurately as possible.

TABLE 16.3. PROMINENT CLINICAL FINDINGS IN PATIENTS WITH HYPERCORTISOLISM

Complications of Excessive Glucocorticoid Exposure	
CARDIOVASCULAR/RENAL	
Atherosclerotic cardiovascular disease	Hypokalemic alkalosis
Hypertension	Sodium and water retention-edema
CENTRAL NERVOUS SYSTEM	
Pseudotumor cerebri	Psychiatric disorders
ENDOCRINE	
Central hypothyroidism	Inhibition of growth hormone secretion
Direct inhibition of growth at epiphysis	Secondary amenorrhea
Elaboration of somatomedin-inhibitory substances	
GASTROINTESTINAL (USUALLY SEEN WITH EXOGENOUS STEROIDS)	
Fatty infiltration of the liver	Pancreatitis
Gastric hemorrhage	Peptic ulceration
Intestinal perforation	
HEMATOLOGIC	
Lymphocytopenia with destruction of lymphoid tissues	Suppression of immune response leading to opportunistic infections
Neutrocytophilia	
INHIBITION OF FIBROPLASIA	
Impaired wound healing	Subcutaneous tissue atrophy
MUSCULOSKELETAL	
Aseptic necrosis of bone	Osteoporosis-vertebral compression fractures
Myopathy	
METABOLIC	
Cushingoid habitus	Insulin-resistant diabetes mellitus
Hyperhidrosis	Negative calcium balance and abnormal vitamin D metabolism
Hyperlipidemia, hypercholesterolemia	
OPHTHALMOLOGIC	
Glaucoma	Posterior subcapsular cataracts

Adapted from Yanovski JA and Cutler GB Jr. Glucocorticoid action and the clinical features of Cushing's syndrome. *Endocrinol Metab Clin North Am* 1994 Sep;23(3):487–509, with permission. Drs. Yanovsky and Cutler had previously adapted the table from Melby JC. Clinical pharmacology of systemic corticosteroids. *Ann Rev Pharmacol and Toxicol* 1977;17:511–527; and Davis GF. Adverse effects of corticosteroids II. Systemic. *Clin Dermatol* 1986;4:161–169, with permission.

Marginally. Obese people eat marginally too much, that is, they eat about fifty-three weeks' worth of food every fifty-two weeks. The systolic blood pressure of hypertensive patients increases marginally—about 1 or 2 mm Hg per year. The blood glucose levels of patients with insulin resistance increase marginally—about 1 or 2 mg/dL per year. The excess glucocorticoid activity required to cause these disorders is on this same small scale, and that is one reason why it has been overlooked for so long.

As was shown in Figure 15.1, cortisol levels are maintained by twin negative feedback loops in the hypothalamic-pituitary-adrenal (HPA) axis. This system is so finely regulated that pituitary and adrenal tumors will not cause large changes in cortisol production unless the tumors are relatively large. Still, like any complex system, the HPA axis makes errors, and these errors become larger with age and stress. When these errors result in supraoptimal cortisol levels, patients gradually develop the symptoms associated with potbelly syndrome.

Supraoptimal. An optimal level of glucocorticoid activity would be one that was:

- high enough to provide appropriate counterregulatory opposition to insulin, but not so high that it would cause chronic insulin resistance.
- high enough to give us a hearty appetite, but not so high that it would make us eat too much.
- high enough to ensure the deposition of appropriate amounts of fat, but not so high that it would make us obese.
- high enough to maintain a normal blood pressure, but not so high that it would make us hypertensive.
- high enough to protect self-cells from the immune system, but not so high that it would protect germs and cancer cells.

As a practical matter, it is impossible to know what the optimal level of glucocorticoid activity is for a particular patient. It is possible, however, to know whether a patient's glucocorticoid activity has been chronically high or low, and we learn this by looking at the signs and symptoms exhibited by the patient, not by checking his or her glucocorticoid levels.

Glucocorticoid. Cortisol is the hormone of greatest interest, but corticosterone and other endogenous and exogenous steroids have effects on metabolism. Cortisone, which appears to have little direct effect on metabolism, is readily converted to cortisol by fat cells.

Activity. I've used the term "activity" instead of "level" because activity is determined by the kind and level of glucocorticoid, and by the patient's sensitivity to the glucocorticoid. Supraoptimal glucocorticoid activity may be caused by any combination of the following conditions:

- Overuse of cortisol-like medicines (the easiest condition to identify and correct).
- Hypersecretion of cortisol. The following conditions have been associated with increased cortisol secretion and are often mentioned in medical textbooks: stress, infections, tumors, obesity, mental depressive disease, alcoholism, anorexia/bulimia nervosa, and the gradual desensitization of the glucocorticoid receptors in the hypothalamus.
- Hypersensitivity of tissues to cortisol. Sensitivity to glucocorticoids varies greatly from person-to-person and it is difficult to measure outside of a few research laboratories.
- Excessive reconversion of cortisone to cortisol by visceral fat (discussed below).

Glucocorticoid activity must be inferred from its effects since there is no way to measure it yet. The most easily diagnosed effect of excess glucocorticoid activity is the accumulation of visceral fat.

VISCERAL FAT

Potbellies are depots for two very distinctive kinds of fat. Subcutaneous fat is located outside of the abdominal muscles—this is the fat that you can squeeze between your fingers. Visceral fat is located inside the abdominal cavity, where it cushions and warms our internal organs. It is this internal fat that is such an important factor in every current version of the dysmetabolic syndrome.[15,16,17]

Stimulated by cortisol, the enlarged abdominal fat store leads to an increased delivery of free fatty acids, which travel directly to the liver through the portal vein. Oxidized free fatty acids block insulin receptors in the liver and make it insulin resistant. Normally, the liver uses 75 percent of the insulin produced by the pancreas. When the liver is insulin resistant, it cannot use as much insulin, with the result that:

- The insulin effect on the liver deteriorates and glucose and lipid levels in the body rise.
- Unused insulin leaves the liver, exposing tissues throughout the body to abnormally high levels of the hormone.
- Free fatty acids infiltrate into the liver itself, resulting in hepatic steatosis.

Cortisol by itself also contributes to the insulin resistance of the liver. The kidneys and colon convert some cortisol to cortisone. Visceral fat reconverts cortisone back to cortisol, and cortisol-laden blood exiting from the visceral fat is fed directly into the liver via the portal vein. The amount of extra cortisol produced by visceral fat is not enough to raise peripheral cortisol levels very much, but it is enough to make the liver insulin resistant. In the liver, cortisol counteracts the effects of insulin on glucose and lipid metabolism, thereby contributing to the elevation of glucose, lipids, and insulin in peripheral blood, as described above.

Cortisol, insulin, and visceral fat create an endless fat-to-fat loop that operates as follows:

1. Cortisol and insulin stimulate the accumulation of visceral fat.
2. Visceral fat produces free fatty acids that flow directly into the liver via the portal vein.
3. Oxidized free fatty acids (and cortisol) produce insulin resistance in the liver.
4. Insulin resistance in the liver raises glucose levels in peripheral tissues.
5. Insulin that should have been metabolized in the liver floods peripheral tissues.
6. The excess insulin contributes to the acummulation of subcutaneous and visceral fat.
7. Return to step 1.

By these mechanisms, insulin resistance, hyperinsulinemia and eventually type 2 diabetes develop. The insulin resistance and/or hyperinsulinemia can in turn generate hypertension by making blood vessels more prone to contract.

If the fat-to-fat theory described above is correct—and there is a lot of evidence to indicate that it is—then cortisol and visceral fat can be seen as the starting points for the cascade of other aberrations and symptoms associated with insulin resistance. Since it is very difficult to evaluate cortisol measurements, visceral fat mass becomes, by default, the most important single factor in diagnosing chronic subtle hypercortisolism.

Since it is very difficult to evaluate cortisol measurements, visceral fat mass becomes, by default, the most important single factor in diagnosing chronic subtle hypercortisolism.

The best way to determine whether a patient has excessive visceral fat is to measure his or her abdominal sagittal diameter (ASD). ASD is defined as the distance from the back, in the supine position, to the highest level of the abdomen. The rationale for using ASD as an indicator of the amount of visceral fat is shown in Figure 16.1, which illustrates two very different types of abdominal fat accumulation.

The illustration on the left represents a person whose obesity is caused primarily by subcutaneous fat. This fat is not bound by the abdominal muscles and it tends to flow out to the sides when the patient is lying on his back.

In the illustration on the right, the abdominal muscles behave like a balloon, compressing visceral fat into a round shape that produces a relatively high ASD measurement. Consequently, ASD is a better indicator of visceral fat mass than either waist size or WHR.

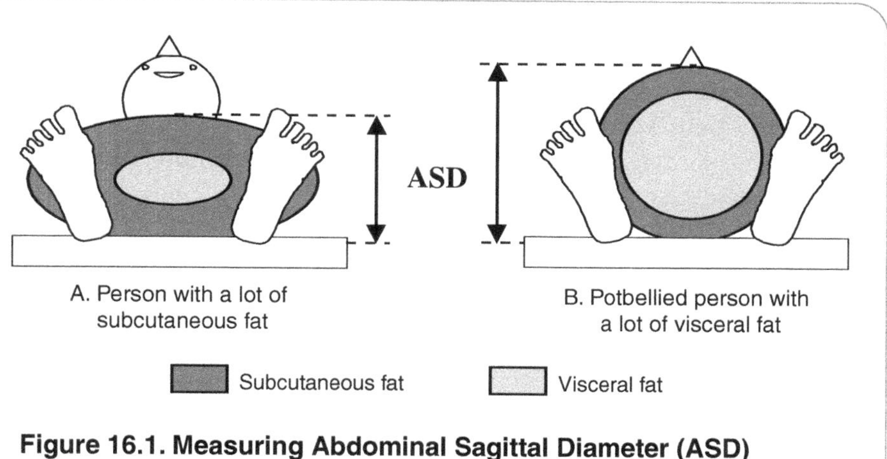

Figure 16.1. Measuring Abdominal Sagittal Diameter (ASD)

Subcutaneous fat tends to flow out to the sides of a patient when he lies on his back, thus reducing his sagittal diameter. The abdominal muscles tend to compress visceral fat into a rounder shape. Consequently, two people with the same waist circumference may have very different sagittal diameters.

ASD has been shown to be a useful clinical marker for dysmetabolic syndromes and it is a better statistical predictor for cardiovascular disease than WHR or obesity.[18]

DIAGNOSING CHRONIC SUBTLE HYPERCORTISOLISM

It is difficult to measure glucocorticoid activity, but it is easy to measure the long-term effects of that activity. Consequently, the diagnosis of chronic subtle hypercortisolism has little or nothing to do with glucocorticoid measurements. In order to judge whether or not a person is suffering from subtle hypercortisolism, the physician must rely on clinical signs and symptoms.

The first diagnostic step is to use Checklist 16.1 to determine whether or not the visceral fat mass is significantly increased. If the visceral fat mass is large, then examine the patient for the secondary markers listed in Checklist 16.2.

If the patient is viscerally obese and has one or more of the secondary markers listed in Checklist 16.2, then it can be assumed that he or she has chronic subtle hypercortisolism.

Cortisol measurements. Measurements of cortisol levels cannot be used to identify subtle hypercortisolism, but they are still valuable. Once you have determined that a patient meets the criteria for a diagnosis of chronic subtle hypercortisolism, the patient should be tested to ensure that he or she does not have a more severe form of hypercortisolism. Cushing's syndrome, for example, resembles type 2 diabetes so closely that it will sometimes remain undiagnosed until the patient dies from it.

Tests for diagnosing severe hypercortisolism are described in many standard medical texts.

CAUSES OF CHRONIC SUBTLE HYPERCORTISOLISM

When you have decided that a patient has chronic subtle hypercortisolism, the next question is "What caused it?" The most common causes are:

- Small tumors, especially adrenal incidentalomas
- Environmental stressors
- Psychiatric or psychological disorders
- Sleep disturbances

Checklist 16.1. Primary Markers for Chronic Subtle Hypercortisolism

Visceral fat mass ☐

Determined by any one of the following methods

a. Abdominal sagittal diameter (ASD) of >10 inches (25 cm) in men or women (preferred method)

b. Waist circumference: > 40 inches (102 cm) for men, or > 35 inches (88 cm) for women, or

c. Waist/hip ratio (WHR): > 0.9 for males or > 0.85 for females

Note: BMI should not be considered when diagnosing PBS.

Checklist 16.2. Secondary Markers for Chronic Subtle Hypercortisolism

1. Hepatic steatosis ☐

Indicated by slight to moderate elevation of alanine aminotransferase (ALT) *and* aspartate transaminase (AST).

Typically, ALT and AST are elevated in parallel, ALT often a little more than AST. These values can of course be elevated for reasons other than hypercortisolism and should not be used in cases of high alcohol consumption.

2. Type 2 diabetes ☐

3. Impaired glucose regulation ☐

a. Fasting blood glucose ≥ 110 mg/dL or

b. Blood glucose ≥ 120 mg/dL 2 hours after a standard 75 g glucose load

4. Insulin resistance ☐

a. Indirectly indicated by a fasting plasma insulin > 12 mU/L, or

b. Insulin resistance as measured by glucose clamp as defined by the local laboratory performing the test

5. Dyslipidemia ☐

a. Plasma triglycerides ≥ 1.7 mmol/L (≥ 150 mg/dL) or

b. Low HDL-cholesterol: < 1.0 mmol/L (< 40 mg/dL) in men; < 1.3 mmol/L (< 50 mg/dL) in women

6. Hypertension ☐

Blood pressure > 130/85 mm Hg

7. Albumin leakage in urine (microalbuminuria) ☐

a. Urinary albumin excretion rate ≥ 20 µg/minute or

b. Albumin/creatinine ratio ≥ 20 mg/g

- Physical ailments such as ischemic lesions and arthritis
- Infections
- Feedback errors in the HPA axis caused by age or disease

The chances are very good that you will never know what is causing the hypercortisolism. Nonetheless, there is quite a bit that can be done to treat it.

TREATING CHRONIC SUBTLE HYPERCORTISOLISM

The first and safest—but not necessarily the most successful—measure is to encourage the patient to minimize the environmental stressors in his or her life. Patients should be encouraged to:

- Organize and manage their lives to minimize everyday stresses.
- Avoid all kinds of agents known to cause harmful stress stimulus to the brain. One of the most powerful and dangerous agents here is alcohol. People who drink too much should contact Alcoholics Anonymous or similar groups. Avoid nicotine and street drugs.
- Minimize the use of prescription drugs, including narcotics, anxiolytics, and sleeping pills, that may affect cortisol production or sensitivity.

It is easy to see the necessity for avoiding stress, alcohol, nicotine, etc., but it is very difficult for people to change their habits, and many people seem to be addicted to stress. Here are some other things to try:

- Mental depression, if present, must be dealt with since this condition is known to be a strong stimulator of cortisol secretion. Alcohol abuse, of course, contributes powerfully to depressive disease.
- Sleep disorders are common and difficult to treat in people with hypercortisolism. Alcohol, stress, and depression interfere with sleep. Patients get caught in a vicious cycle because cortisol interferes with sleep, and lack of sleep raises cortisol levels. Breaking this cycle is difficult and time consuming. Avoid sleep-inducing drugs, and help patients who are using these drugs get free of them.
- It is well known that physical activity counteracts virtually all known risk factors for cardiovascular disease and type 2 diabetes. At least some of this benefit may be derived from cortisol reduction because any enjoy-

able physical activity that does not injure tissues will counteract cortisol secretion. Walking an hour every day is better than running or other types of hard exercise once or twice per week.

There are more suggestions in Chapters 18 through 20 for dealing with subtle hypercortisolism.

SUMMARY

Since the medical world is still largely unaware of cortisol's role in insulin resistance, obesity, type 2 diabetes, and hypertension, these disorders are often blamed on (1) a disproportionately high intake of calories and (2) insufficient physical activity.

People suffering from chronic subtle hypercortisolism—potbelly syndrome—are therefore often told to eat less and exercise more in order to recover. However, the prognoses for such measures are unfortunately very poor. The most discouraging consequence of this is that the affected person is blamed for his or her own condition. In most cases, this is deeply unfair.

A more widespread understanding and acceptance of the role of cortisol in the development of potbellies and related illnesses would change this situation dramatically in the future. Although specific treatments aimed at normalizing elevated cortisol activity in patients with the potbelly syndrome, Syndrome X, and dysmetabolic syndrome are still not generally accepted in the medical community, I am convinced that this is only a matter of time.

REFERENCES

Epigraph: Prevalence among U.S. Adults of a Metabolic Syndrome Associated with Obesity. Findings from the Third NHANES Survey. National Center for Chronic Disease Prevention and Health Promotion, Centers for Disease Control.

1. Kretschmer E. *Körperbau und Charakter.* Berlin: Springer, 1921.

2. Gaisböck F. Die polycythemia. *Ergeb Inn Med Kinderheilkd* 1922;21:210.

3. Vague J. La differenciation sexuelle facteur determinant des formes de l'obesit. *Press Med* 1947;55:339–341.

4. Krotkiewski M, Butruk E, Zembrzuska Z. Les fonctions corticosurrenales dans les divers types morphologiques d'obesité. *Le Diabète* 1966;19:229–233.

5. Herberg L, Bergmann M, Hennigs U, et al. Influence of diet on the metabolic syndrome of obesity. *Isr J Med Sci* 1972;8:822–823.

6. Reaven GH. Role of insulin resistance in human disease. *Diabetes* 1988;37: 1595–1607.

7. Definition, Diagnosis and Classification of Diabetes Mellitus and Its Complications. *Report of a WHO Consultation.* Part 1: Diagnosis and Classification of Diabetes Mellitus. World Health Organization Department of Noncommunicable Disease Surveillance, Geneva, 1998.

8. National Institutes of Health. 2001 May. ATP III At-A-Glance: Quick Desk Reference. NIH Publication No. 01-3305.

9. Mårin P, Darin N, Amemiya T, et al. P. Cortisol secretion in relation to body fat distribution in obese premenopausal women. *Metabolism* 1992;41:882–886.

10. Pasquali R, Cantobelli S, Casimirri F, et al. The hypothalamo-pituitary-adrenal axis in obese women with different patterns of body fat distribution. *J Clin Endocrinol Metab* 1993;77:341–346.

11. Ljung T, Andersson B, Björntorp P, and Mårin P. Inhibition of cortisol secretion by dexamethason in relation to body fat distribution, a dose-response study. *Obes Res* 1996;4:277–282.

12. Marniemi J, Kronholm E, Aunola S, et al. Visceral fat and psychosocial stress in identical twins discordant for obesity. *J Intern Med* 2002;251(1):35–43.

13. Rosmond R and Bjorntorp P. Low cortisol production in chronic stress. The connection stress-somatic disease is a challenge for future research. *Lakartidningen* 2000;97(38):4120–4124.

14. Björntorp P and Rosmond R. Neuroendocrine abnormalities in visceral obesity. *Int J Obes Relat Metab Disord* 2000;24 Suppl 2:S80–S85.

15. Fujioka S, Matsuzawa Y, Tokunaga K, et al. Contribution of intra-abdominal fat accumulation to the impairment of glucose and lipid metabolism in human obesity. *Metabolism* 1987;36:54–59.

16. Haffner SM. Obesity and the metabolic syndrome: The San Antonio Heart Study. *Br J Nutr* 2000;83 Suppl 1:S67–S70.

17. Arner P. Insulin resistance in type 2 diabetes: Role of fatty acids. *Diabetes Metab Res Rev* 2002;18 Suppl 2:S5–S9.

18. Kumlin L, Dimberg L, and Mårin P. Ratio of abdominal sagittal diameter to height is strong indicator of coronary risk. *BMJ* 1997;314:830.

Taking Charge of Your Own Health

Translation of research findings into sustainable improvements in clinical outcomes and patient outcomes remains a substantial obstacle to improving the quality of care. Up to two decades may pass before the findings of original research becomes part of routine clinical practice.

—TRANSLATING RESEARCH INTO PRACTICE (TRIP)-II
U.S. AGENCY FOR HEALTHCARE RESEARCH AND QUALITY

Research findings are like pieces of a jigsaw puzzle—piece X is not very interesting until it is joined to its neighbors and a pattern emerges. If the neighboring pieces are missing, they have to be found first, and joined to piece X, before X adds to our understanding of the big picture.

The obesity, diabetes, and heart disease puzzle couldn't be solved until recently because too many pieces were missing. Now that we know more about infections and cortisol, a clear pattern has emerged. The picture is not complete yet, but when it is complete it will look very similar to the infection-cortisol model of chronic illness shown in Figure 17.1.

Your doctor, regardless of her specialty, will be familiar with every element in Figure 17.1, but she is not likely to understand them well enough to see how each one leads to the next. Consequently, and understandably, she is unlikely to believe that she can treat obesity by treating infections. Until you find a doctor who understands the chain of events leading from infections to your health problem, you will have to rely on your own knowledge and initiative to stay well. This chapter provides some general information about taking care of yourself, and the next two chapters provide details.

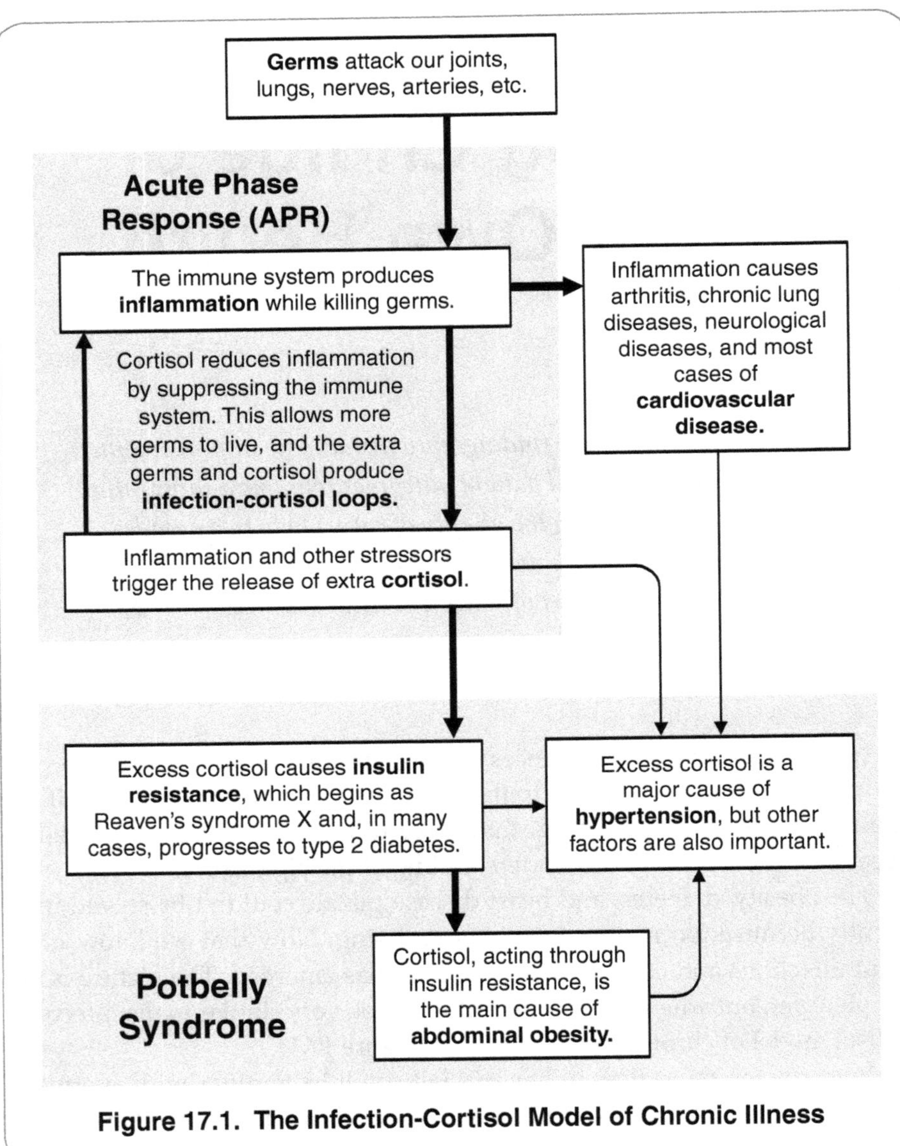

Figure 17.1. The Infection-Cortisol Model of Chronic Illness

DO YOUR OWN RESEARCH

Your germs, your immune system, and your symptoms are not like anyon else's. Figuring out exactly what ails you can take a lot of time and effort, s you can't expect your doctor to do all of it by herself.

Anyone with access to the Internet can become a medical researcher. When I have a question about something, I begin my search for an answer by "googling." To "google" something, go to Google's advanced search engine (www.google.com/advanced_search). Type in the words or phrases you are interested in, set the conditions for the search, and then click on "search." With practice, you can learn an amazing amount of useful information by "googling."

A nice feature of Google's advanced search engine is that you can restrict your searches to certain Internet "domains." Here are the most important domains, ranked from most reliable to least:

1. Military (.mil). Limited range of subjects. Excellent information on stress.
2. Government (.gov). Best source of medical information.
3. Educational (.edu). The accuracy and clarity of information varies greatly.
4. Organizational (.org). Valuable, but often highly biased.
5. Commercial (.com). Biased and inaccurate, but extensive.

The PubMed website (www.ncbi.nih.gov/entrez/query.fcgi) is invaluable for anyone doing medical research because it provides the abstracts of millions of articles from medical journals. If an abstract is particularly interesting, I drive to a medical library and make a copy of the entire article.

TUTORING YOUR DOCTORS

My doctors know more than I do, but they don't know everything I know, and frequently they do not know things that are important to me (such as the difference between *Chlamydia trachomatis* and *Chlamydophila pneumoniae*). A few years ago, to make sure my doctors knew everything they needed to know about my illnesses, I started tutoring them. They don't like it very much, but their likes and dislikes are not as important as my health. Here's an example of how I tutor the doctors in my giant HMO.

After my heart attack, I asked to be tested for *Chlamydophila pneumoniae* (CPN). My doctor didn't think the test was necessary, so I wrote several letters explaining why I needed it, supporting my arguments with abstracts from PubMed. After reading the letters, and listening to my lengthy discussions of CPN-related illnesses, my doctor finally ordered the tests. I tested positive, of course, just as most older people will.

After doing more research and writing more letters, I got my doctor to prescribe clarithromycin. That resulted in the short but miraculous recovery described in Chapter 1. Doing all of the research, writing the letters, and arguing with my doctors took five months, but it was time well spent. I still use carefully crafted letters, supported by PubMed abstracts, to twist the arms of my HMO doctors.

Tutoring doctors is a lot of work, and patients with chronic illnesses may not have enough energy to do it. Fortunately, there are some safe ways to reduce your cortisol and boost your energy and spirits. Start with some of the easy things recommended in Chapters 18 and 19, such as watching funny movies and getting massages. These activities will make you feel better without much effort on your part. With luck, you may feel well enough to start training your doctors.

COMPLEMENTARY AND ALTERNATIVE MEDICINE

The things that we can do for ourselves, without prescriptions from doctors, are classified by the NIH as *complementary and alternative medicine* (CAM). The U.S. National Center for Complementary and Alternative Medicine (NCCAM, http://nccam.nih.gov/), defines CAM as:

> Medical and health care systems, practices, and products that are not presently considered to be part of conventional medicine. While some scientific evidence exists regarding some CAM therapies, for most there are key questions that are yet to be answered through well-designed scientific studies—questions such as whether these therapies are safe and whether they work for the diseases or medical conditions for which they are used.

Chapters 18 and 19 discuss CAM therapies that may help you lower cortisol levels. I suggest that you read these chapters, make a list of any "systems, practices, and products" that interest you, and do your own research on them.

KEEP A DIARY

Many CAM therapies work slowly, so it may be hard to know whether they are making you better or worse. If you have a chronic illness, I suggest that you keep a health diary. Record which pills you are taking, how you feel, your blood pressure, and weight. Note how long and how well you sleep because many medications and CAM therapies can keep you awake. Use a highlighter to draw attention to changes in your regimen or your health. Later, you can go over the diary and get a better idea of what worked and what didn't.

A health diary can save you a lot of money—some of the supplements listed in Chapter 19 are expensive, and a diary will help you decide whether they are worth what they cost. Keeping a diary helped me to recognize that vitamin E raises my blood pressure, so I don't take large doses of it now.

YOU CAN KILL GERMS BY AVOIDING STRESS

There is very little that we can do to kill germs directly without the help of a physician. We can, however, kill germs indirectly by avoiding stress.

Chapter 3 described a sequence of events—an infection-cortisol (IC) loop—that facilitates the growth of our old germs and makes us more susceptible to new ones. If we delay any event in an IC loop, we delay all of the subsequent events. To see how this works, let's review the main features of the IC loop:

1. Every day we are exposed to stressors.
2. Our reactions to those stressors may include the release of extra cortisol.
3. The extra cortisol weakens our immune system and makes us more susceptible to infections.
4. Our old infections flare up a little, and occasionally we will get a new infection.
5. The immune system produces more inflammatory cells and cytokines.
6. The inflammatory cytokines trigger the release of extra cortisol.
7. Our health declines a little.
8. Return to event 1.

We have limited control over each event, but we do have some. If we reduce our exposure to stressors in event 1, we will not release as much cortisol in event 2. Increasing our resistance to stress will also reduce the amount of cortisol released in event 2. Any reduction in the amount of cortisol released in event 2 will make us less susceptible to infection in event 3, and that will delay the start of flare-ups or new infections in event 4. Thus avoiding stressors, or improving stress resistance, will slow the operation of the infection-cortisol loop and delay the acquisition of new infections.

Slowing the progression of an illness is desirable, but it is not very inspiring. Fortunately, our efforts can sometimes stop or even reverse our IC loops.

SEMI-SPONTANEOUS REMISSIONS

Avoiding stress usually produces a "linear dose-response relationship." This means that a small decrease in stress produces a small decrease in illness, and a larger decrease in stress produces a larger decrease in illness. Sometimes, however, small stress reductions produce huge improvements in our health. These events are usually called *spontaneous remissions*.

Spontaneous remissions are seldom completely spontaneous. In most cases, there are changes in the attitudes or behaviors of patients who later have remissions. I believe that these semi-spontaneous remissions can be explained by the existence of some kind of "tipping point" in our immune systems. When cortisol levels are above the tipping point, the immune system can kill a few germs, but it can't eradicate them. Consequently, a small reduction in stress and cortisol will produce a small improvement in our health, a phenomenon that has been documented many times.

If a patient's cortisol level is near her immune system's tipping point, then a small reduction in stress may be enough to drop her cortisol level below the tipping point. When that happens, her monocytes, macrophages, and other immune cells "wake up" and start to kill germs much faster than they did before. If her immune cells kill germs fast enough, the IC loop is reversed and it becomes an immunity-health loop. Such a loop would work like this:

1. The patient reduces her stress level.
2. Her cortisol drops a little below her immune system's tipping point.
3. Her immune system kills many more germs.
4. The improvement in immunity is enough to suppress or eradicate one of her infections.
5. Her immune system releases fewer inflammatory cytokines.
6. Her HPA axis produces slightly less cortisol.
7. Her health improves a little.
8. Return to event 1.

An immunity-health loop would eradicate or suppress some infections, but not all, so eventually it would run its course, stop, reverse, and become an infection-cortisol loop again. This sequence of events would produce a typical spontaneous remission experience—a patient suddenly gets well, then her health gradually returns to its previous condition. Her doctor almost never knows what caused the remission, or what ended it.

The recommendations provided in the next three chapters are based on the assumption that it is possible to increase the frequency and duration of semi-spontaneous remissions by reducing stress and fighting infections. If I'm right, you may be able to experience the kind of recovery I described in Chapter 1, and have it last for years instead of months. If I'm wrong, the worst that is likely to happen is that you will experience small improvements in your health proportional to the effort you make.

SUMMARY

For some years to come, you will have a difficult time finding doctors who are interested in middle-path germs or chronic subtle hypercortisolism (pot-belly syndrome). While you are looking for a doctor who knows the difference between *Chlamydophila pneumoniae* and *Chlamydia trachomatis,* you will have to do your own research, tutor your doctors, and take notes on what works for you and what doesn't. You can slow down, and possibly reverse, the operation of infection-cortisol loops by avoiding stressors (the next chapter) or building up resistance to stress (Chapter 19).

8 Avoiding Stressors

Now I counsel you to make a studied business of relaxing and taking things easy, getting to the office late, taking trips, and making everybody else work like hell. . . .

I woke up at about [the age of] thirty-three to the fact that I was working myself to death, to my superior's advantage, and that I was acquiring the reputation of being merely a pick and shovel man. From that time on, I made it a business to avoid, so far as possible, detail work, and to relax as completely as I could manage in a pleasurable fashion.

—Advice given by General George C. Marshall to a newly appointed general

General Marshall rode his horse each morning, then went to work when he felt like it. He took a nap after lunch, and he almost never worked later than 4:00 P.M. In the evenings, when his subordinates were still at work, he took long walks with his wife.

Between his morning rides, afternoon naps, and evening walks, General Marshall found time to oversee the winning of World War II, create the Marshall Plan that rebuilt Europe, serve as secretary of state, write several books, and win the Nobel Peace Prize in 1953.

General Marshall was able to accomplish so much *because* of his work habits, not *despite* them. He took good care of his mind and body, and, in his own words, he tried to "save [his] ammunition for the big fights and avoid a constant drain of little ones."[1] The small fights that he avoided were stressors that most of us take for granted: keeping our nose to the grindstone, not getting enough sleep, and worrying about trivial details.

In this chapter we will look at several ways of emulating General Marshall by avoiding small stressors.

KINDS OF STRESS

Stressors can be divided broadly into five categories: psychosocial, environmental, physiological, cognitive, and emotional. Within those categories, stressors can be further divided into: internal, external, background, or transient. Table 18.1 lists a few examples from each category.[2]

Notice that many of the stressors listed in Table 18.1 are also stress responses, so it is easy to get ourselves tangled in long chains of stressors. For example, the additional stress of air travel when we are fatigued may lead to an infection that causes inflammation and pain that cause sleeplessness. All six stressors raise cortisol levels.

TABLE 18.1. COMMON STRESSORS

	Usual Source			
Stressors	**Internal**	**External**	**Background**	**Transient**
PSYCHOSOCIAL STRESSORS				
Living beyond our means	■		■	
Difficult job, or no job		■	■	
Family problems		■	■	
Mean, rude, or scary people		■		■
ENVIRONMENTAL STRESSORS				
Chronic infections		■	■	
Television		■	■	
Excessive heat or cold		■	■	
Taxes and other natural disasters		■	■	
Acute infections		■	■	
Alcohol, caffeine, nicotine, sugar		■	■	
Travel, especially by air		■		■
High altitude (hypoxia)		■		■
Uncomfortable or scary places		■		■
Noise, traffic, air pollution		■		■

Stressors	Usual Source: Internal	Usual Source: External	Background	Transient
PHYSIOLOGICAL STRESSORS				
Breathing problems (hypoxia)	■		■	
Acute phase responses	■		■	
Inflammation from any source	■		■	
Sleeplessness, exhaustion, fatigue	■		■	
Pain	■		■	
Hunger, thirst, low blood sugar	■			■
COGNITIVE STRESSORS				
Worry	■		■	
Conflicting obligations	■		■	
Frustration	■		■	
Catastrophizing (scaring oneself)	■		■	
EMOTIONAL STRESSORS				
Anxiety, cynicism, fear, hostility	■		■	
Loneliness, unrequited love	■		■	
Low self-esteem	■		■	

Some stressors are more pleasant than others, and by indulging in the pleasant stressors we can kick our cortisol levels up so high, and numb ourselves so much, that we can tolerate the unpleasant stressors. This often leads to stressor-stressor loops that destroy our health and happiness. The most common stressor-stressor loop is drinking coffee to stay alert at work or school. The caffeine interferes with our sleep, so we wake up tired. We need coffee to wake up, and more coffee to stay awake. The caffeine and sleeplessness both raise our cortisol levels, and cortisol interferes with sleep. This coffee-sleeplessness-cortisol loop makes us more susceptible to infections, heart disease, and potbelly syndrome.

Trying to untangle stressor chains and loops is beyond the scope of this book, but the next few pages suggest ways to avoid some stressors.

AVOIDING EXTERNAL STRESSORS

Most literature on stress focuses on avoiding external stressors because they are easy to recognize. The following excerpt from an NIH pamphlet is typical:

> First try to identify the things in your life that cause you stress: marital problems, conflict at work, a death or illness in the family. Once you identify and understand how these stressors affect you, you can begin to figure out ways to change your environment and manage them. If there's a problem that can be solved, set about taking control and solving it. For example, you might decide to change jobs if problems at work are making you too stressed.[3]

That is good advice, but don't get divorced or quit your job too soon. People who are heavily stressed are often distracted or depressed, and it is hard for them to rationally analyze the source of their problems, make wise decisions, and then follow through with an appropriate course of action. Still, unless you are completely overwhelmed by illness or stress, there are many things you can do to avoid stressors. Make a list of things that bug you, then cross out the ones that you absolutely cannot do anything about. Then start working on the problems you can fix. Don't try to solve all of them at once, and start with small ones for practice. Think positively, and avoid extreme solutions to simple problems.

A few external stressors are described below. Except for air travel, they are all easy to avoid (unless you are addicted to them).

Air travel. The effect of a stressor on our health is determined by how stressful it is and how long we are exposed to it. Air travel is stressful, even for people who love it, but the stress is not likely to harm us unless we fly frequently and don't get enough rest between trips. Flying from west to east is more stressful than flying the other way, so people traveling from west to east ought to give themselves extra time to rest and relax at their destinations.[4]

Alcohol. This common stressor raises our cortisol levels and disrupts our diurnal cycles, producing many of the unpleasant effects of jet lag even if we haven't been near a jet.[5]

Caffeine. Caffeine is an alkaloid poison produced by several plants to protect themselves from insects. Drinking this poison floods your body with stress hormones. The hormones make you feel alert and on top of things for a while, then, as the hormones wear off, you feel listless and tired. Feeling tired becomes a signal to drink another cup of bug poison to counteract the effects of the last cup. Caffeine raises cortisol levels and blood pressure directly, and it makes you more sensitive to other stressors.[6,7]

Recent studies have suggested that coffee, tea, and chocolate are good for some people. Unless you are sure that you are one of those people who benefit from drinking bug poison, you should probably avoid it.

Cold. I once got the brilliant idea that swimming in cold water would help me burn more calories and lose weight. I was wrong. Being cold raises our cortisol levels, and the result is that we gain weight instead of losing it.

Nicotine. Nicotine is one of several bug poisons produced by tobacco plants. When we smoke, these poisons trigger the release of cortisol. Nicotine has different effects on men versus women, on the lean versus the fat, and on new versus habitual users. Secondhand smoke, for example, kicks cortisol levels higher in nonsmokers than firsthand smoke does in habitual smokers. Think about that the next time you light up near other people.

Smoking desensitizes cortisol-regulating systems so much that smokers cannot always produce enough cortisol to protect themselves during a crisis. Consequently, they have a lower chance of surviving accidents or serious infections.

Noise. Loud music raises the cortisol levels of animals and humans,[8,9] and the ordinary traffic sounds found in small towns can increase the cortisol levels of children.[10] Noise is also a risk factor for heart attacks. German researchers found that long exposure to moderately high noise, roughly the same noise level you would find in a noisy office, greatly increases the likelihood that men, but not women, will have heart attacks.[11]

Sugar. It is often hard to identify stressors, so some researchers argue that any particular item or experience is a stressor for person X if, and only if, it raises the cortisol level of person X. Using this standard, plain table sugar (sucrose) may be an important stressor.

In his 1972 book, *Sweet and Dangerous,* John Yudkin described an experiment in which he and his colleagues measured the cortisol levels of eleven volunteers before putting them on a high-sugar diet for two weeks. At the end of the experiment, the cortisol levels of the volunteers were three to four times as high as they had been at the beginning.[12]

Until you actually try to avoid sugar, it seems like giving it up would be an easy task. The truth is that sugar is very difficult to avoid. It is used to sweeten and "bulk up" hundreds of common food items, so you may be eating a lot of sugar even if you never add it to your breakfast cereal.

BANISH YOUR TELEVISION

Television is an insidious and pervasive stressor. The programs are designed to make us sit through commercials, and the commercials are designed to make us feel helpless, ugly, smelly, and stupid unless we buy the products being touted.

Why do we watch television when it is so obviously against our best interests? I think we do it for the same reason we do lots of dumb things—it's exciting. John Logan, my old yoga teacher, once said that everyone intuitively knows how to live a healthy, happy life, but when forced to make a choice, most of us will choose excitement over health and happiness. Caffeine, cocaine, nicotine, and television all simultaneously excite and numb us, and they all increase cortisol production.

Do you remember the lovely Miss Meribelle from the dieting thought experiment? Imagine her as an active, fun-loving girl growing up on a remote ranch without television. She is tall and willowy and she weighs 125 pounds. Her systolic blood pressure is 100 and her HPA axis produces 20 pulses of cortisol a day—typical for a healthy young adult. Imagine further that she moves to San Diego at the age of twenty and buys her first television. For two or three hours a day—hours that she might have spent dancing or entertaining friends—she sits and allows herself to be assaulted by the hucksters who write commercials and the cretins who produce TV programs.

Every night she witnesses a parade of real and imagined horrors worse than our grandparents were likely to see in a lifetime. Her higher brain centers will filter out most of this garbage, but some of it will leak down into her hypothalamus. The hypothalamus can't distinguish between real and phony stresses very well, so Miss Meribelle's hypothalamus will be tricked into releasing extra pulses of cortisol. This is a thought experiment, not a real one, so we can't say for sure how many extra pulses she will produce. Let's be conservative and guess that she averages one extra pulse of cortisol a day. This increases her exposure to cortisol by a modest 5 percent. Most of this extra cortisol will be produced in the evenings, when her cortisol levels should be dropping. Consequently, the extra cortisol produced by television will have much larger negative effects on her sleep, appetite, fat storage, and blood pressure than the same amount of extra cortisol would have produced earlier in the day.

We don't know how much this small increase in cortisol will increase her weight and blood pressure, so let's continue to be conservative and guess that they will both increase by 1 percent per year. When she is forty, Miss Meribelle will weigh 153 pounds. Her blood pressure will be 122, which ome experts now consider to be hypertensive. Ten years later, she will weigh 68 pounds and her blood pressure will be 135.

The increased weight and blood pressure are just the twin tips of the roverbial iceberg. Miss Meribelle will be insulin resistant and she will have dozen or more cortisol-related health problems. She will be more anxious, epressed, and friendless than she would have been without television. Her mmune system will be suppressed so she will have more infections. Exercise vill be painful, and she will watch more and more television as her condition eteriorates.

Does this sound far-fetched? Maybe it is, but researchers from California eported that watching television was associated with poor education, low ncome, physical inactivity, alcohol abuse, obesity, high levels of hostility, and epression.[13] All seven of these characteristics are risk factors for heart disase, and they are all linked to excess cortisol.

If you can't give up television—and few people can—then banish it to the nost remote and uncomfortable part of your home. Then, you can watch nything that you really need to see, but you will be less tempted to become couch potato.

VOIDING INTERNAL STRESSORS

ven if you arrange to live an idyllic life free from television and other exteral stressors, you won't be happy or healthy if your brain is full of stressful deas and emotions. A few of the most common internal stressors are disussed below.

atastrophizing. Years ago I drove past some power lines near the end of an irport runway. I got to thinking about how dumb it was to put power lines here, and soon I was wondering what would happen if a small plane hit the vires. In another minute, my imaginary plane was on fire and the passengers vere begging me to save them! By now I had a white-knuckled death grip on ny steering wheel and I was as tense as if I were trapped in the plane myself. t took me a couple of minutes to calm down and start breathing normally gain.

Catastrophizing—imagining awful things and worrying about how we vould deal with them—may have had survival value for our ancestors, who ived much more dangerous lives than we do. It may still be a valuable habit or soldiers and others in dangerous jobs. For most of us, however, catastrohizing is a bad habit that raises our cortisol levels unnecessarily.

An article written for the May/June 1994 issue of *Psychology Toda* discusses ways of recognizing and dealing with this problem. The article i entitled "Avoiding Catastrophic Thinking," and it can be downloaded fron http://cms.psychologytoday.com/articles/pto-19940501-000020.html.

Hostility. Researchers from the University of Utah found that hostile me secreted twice as much cortisol during the day as nonhostile men.[14] Thei findings may explain why hostile people tend to suffer from many illnesse especially cardiovascular diseases.

It is much easier to recognize hostility in other people than it is to see it i ourselves. Still, we can spot examples of our own hostility if we try. If you ar never happy with the service you get in restaurants, or you frequently honl your horn at the idiots in front of you, or you yell at your television, then yo may have a hostile personality.

If you think you might have a hostility problem, I suggest that you rea *The U.S. Army War College Guide to Executive Health and Fitness,* and pay par ticular attention to Chapters 3 and 5. The guide can be downloaded fron www.cdc.gov/nccdphp/dnpa/usphs/pdfs/army.pdf.

Low self-esteem. It makes sense that people with a high sense of self-esteen will feel more capable of handling challenges than will people with low self esteem. Following from that, we would expect people with high self-esteen to experience less stress when performing difficult tasks than would peopl with low self-esteem. To find out whether this theory is true, researchers fron Yale University performed an interesting experiment. First, they tested six teen healthy senior citizens to measure their self-esteem. Next, they meas ured their cortisol levels. Then, they exposed the subjects to simulate driving stresses and measured their cortisol levels again.[15] Not surprisingly the people with the lowest self-esteem had the largest increases in cortisol.

Like most internal stressors, low self-esteem is not glaringly obviou to the people who are suffering from it. According to an article on the websit of the U.S. National Mental Health Information Center (NMHIC), you ma have a problem with low self-esteem if you find yourself frequently repeatin negative messages about yourself:

> Once you have learned them, you may have repeated these negative messages over and over to yourself, especially when you were not feeling well or when you were having a hard time. You may have come to believe them. You may have even worsened the problem by making up some negative

messages or thoughts of your own. These negative thoughts or messages make you feel bad about yourself and lower your self-esteem.[16]

The NMHIC article is entitled *Building Self-esteem: A Self-Help Guide.* It focuses on helping people with self-esteem problems, but it contains valuable advice for anyone who is trying to deal with internal stressors. The article can be downloaded from www.mentalhealth.samhsa.gov/publications/allpubs/SMA-3715/default.asp.

Pain. Pain is one of the clearest signs that something bad is happening to us, and it is a powerful stressor. Danish researchers measured the cortisol levels of ten healthy male volunteers. The volunteers then gave themselves painful electrical shocks for thirty minutes, after which the researchers measured their cortisol levels again.[17] After the self-inflicted shocks, cortisol levels increased two- to threefold.

If you are looking for ways to manage pain, I suggest that you start with the *NINDS Chronic Pain Information Page,* a website maintained by the U.S. National Institute of Neurological Disorders and Stroke. It provides links to organizations that are devoted to eliminating pain, and it also provides links to pain-related publications. *The NINDS Chronic Pain Information Page* website can be found at www.ninds.nih.gov/disorders/chronic_pain/chronic_pain.htm.

SUMMARY

There are many kinds of stressors, but we have only a limited number of ways of coping with them. We can eliminate them, avoid them, or live with them. If we live with them, we have to adapt to them, and the most common adaptation is a chronic increase in our cortisol levels. The extra cortisol numbs us and allows us to continue our everyday activities for many years, but the extra cortisol also causes potbelly syndrome and contributes to heart disease.

Internal stressors are difficult to identify. I became a chronic catastrophizer when I was a nineteen-year-old Navy aircrewman, and I didn't realize what I was doing until forty years later. There are no simple, quick ways to eliminate or avoid internal stressors. I try to catch myself getting anxious or angry about silly things, and then I bring myself back down to a calmer mood. I walk around my neighborhood and chat with people, and I do the breathing exercises I learned in a yoga class. Yoga and other methods of coping with stress are discussed in the next chapter.

RECOMMENDED READING AND RESOURCES

A Guide for Senior Leaders: Stress and the Mind-Body Connection, by Paul T. Harig.

The armed forces have a great interest in controlling stress, and military (.mil) websites contain clearly written practical information on this topic. Colonel Harig's article is excellent, especially the account of General Marshall's work habits. The article can be downloaded from: http://hooah4health.com/mind/stressmgmt/stressmindbody5.htm.

Caffeine Blues: Wake Up to the Hidden Dangers of America's #1 Drug, by Stephen Cherniske (Warner Books, 1998).

Caffeine is an addictive poison. You will sleep better, look better, work better, play better, and be a lot more lovable if you follow the advice given in this book.

Chicken Soup for the Soul: Living Your Dreams, by Jack Canfield and Mark Victor Hansen (HCI, 2003).

These stories are good for you.

Is It Worth Dying For?: How to Make Stress Work for You—Not against You, by Dr. Robert S. Eliot and Dennis L. Breo (Bantam, 1989).

The first part of this book is an excellent description of the dangers of stress, and there are a lot of useful tips for identifying and reducing it. The second half of the book is not as useful.

REFERENCES

Epigraph: Quoted in Harig PT. A Guide for Senior Leaders: Stress and the Mind-Body Connection. http://hooah4health.com/mind/stressmgmt/stressmindbody5.htm.

1. Harig PT. A Guide for Senior Leaders: Stress and the Mind-Body Connection. http://hooah4health.com/mind/stressmgmt/stressmindbody5.htm

2. Office of the Adjutant General, 1st Battalion (GSAB) 140th Aviation Regiment. February 3, 2004. Aeromedical Training: Stress Defined.

Some of the material in this section was adapted from this source.

3. Wein H. A Word to the Wise . . . Stress Control. National Institutes of Health Office of Communications and Public Liaison.

4. O'Connor PJ, Morgan WP, Koltyn KF, et al.. Air travel across four time zones in college swimmers. *J Appl Physiol* 1991 Feb;70(2):756–763.

5. Swift R and Davidson D. Alcohol Hangover Mechanisms and Mediators. *Alcohol Health & Research World* 1998;22(1): 56-60.

6. al'Absi M, Lovallo WR, McKey B, et al. Hypothalamic-pituitary-adrenocortical responses to psychological stress and caffeine in men at high and low risk for hypertension. *Psychosom Med* 1998 Jul-Aug;60(4):521–527.

7. Shepard JD, al'Absi M, Whitsett TL, et al. Additive pressor effects of caffeine and stress in male medical students at risk for hypertension. *Am J Hypertens* 2000 May;13(5 Pt 1):475–481.

8. Gue M, Alvinerie M, Junien JL, et al. Stimulation of kappa opiate receptors in intestinal wall affects stress-induced increase of plasma cortisol in dogs. *Brain Res* 1989 Nov 13;502(1):143–148.

9. Bergomi M, Rovesti S, and Vivoli G. Biological response to noise and other physical stressors in places of entertainment. *Public Health Rev* 1991–92;19(1–4): 263–275.

10. Evans GW, Lercher P, Meis M, et al.. Community noise exposure and stress in children. *J Acoust Soc Am* 2001 Mar;109(3):1023–1027.

11. W Beule, B Schust, M Kersten, et al. Traffic noise and risk of myocardial infarction. *Epidemiology.* 2005 Jan;16(1):33–40.

12. Yudkin, John. *Sweet and Dangerous.* New York: Peter H. Wyden, 1972, p. 109.

13. Sidney S, Sternfeld B, Haskell WL, et al. Television viewing and cardiovascular risk factors in young adults: The CARDIA study. *Ann Epidemiol* 1996 Mar;6(2):154–159.

14. Pope MK and Smith TW. Cortisol excretion in high and low cynically hostile men. *Psychosom Med* 1991 Jul-Aug;53(4):386–392.

15. Seeman TE, Berkman LF, Gulanski BI, et al. Self-esteem and neuroendocrine response to challenge: MacArthur studies of successful aging. *J Psychosom Res* 1995 Jan;39(1):69–84.

16. U.S. National Mental Health Information Center (NMHIC). "Building Self-Esteem: A Self-Help Guide." www.mentalhealth.samhsa.gov/publications/all pubs/SMA-3715/default.asp.

17. Greisen J, Juhl CB, Grofte T, et al. Acute pain induces insulin resistance in humans. *Anesthesiology* 2001 Sep;95(3):578–584.

19 Building Stress Resistance

Research has shown . . . that psychological stress can contribute to increased heart disease and decreased immune system functioning. Other research has demonstrated that cognitions (attitudes, beliefs, values), social support, prayer, and meditation can reduce psychological stress and contribute to positive health outcomes.

—NATIONAL INSTITUTES OF HEALTH (DOCUMENT RFA OB-03-004)

We all have limits to the amount of stress that we can handle and remain healthy. If too much stress is thrust upon us, or we voluntarily take on too much, then we begin to stagger under the load. We look and feel like a half-ton truck hauling a full ton of garbage to the dump.

Alcohol, caffeine, nicotine, sleeping pills, and extra cortisol can help us carry an overload of stress for years, but the extra stress, plus the extra chemicals, will wring the joy out of life and ruin our health. The previous chapter presented ways to avoid stressors. This chapter suggests ways of living, and living well, with the stressors we cannot avoid.

KEEP YOUR HYPOTHALAMUS HAPPY

One of the most enjoyable ways to improve our stress resistance is to look for ways to make our hypothalamus happy. Your hypothalamus is part of your brain, but it isn't the part that figures out whether the world is safe or dangerous, loving or hateful. If your higher brain centers think the world is dangerous and hateful, your hypothalamus will always be on edge, ready to release another dollop of cortisol at the slightest threat or annoyance.

On the other hand, if your higher brain centers think the world is beautiful, safe, fun, and loving, it will take a much larger annoyance to make your hypothalamus release more cortisol. Here are a few things that lower cortisol levels by reassuring your hypothalamus that everything is going to be OK.

Forgive people. A grudge, no matter how justified it may be, is a psychic sore that eats away at you, not the person who injured you. A researcher from Stanford explained it this way:

> When we are particularly angry about an event over a long period of time, there is often a psychological cost in terms of stress, hostility, strained relationships and so forth. But there is a physical cost as well. When we're especially agitated we produce cortisol, a body chemical, which can help us rally and gain brief strength against a threat. However, an elevated level of cortisol for a prolonged period is implicated in several serious diseases, including diabetes, hypertension and cancer.[1]

Calmly and rationally decide whether you want to "get even" with people who have harmed you. If you can't get revenge, or you don't want to get revenge, then forgive and forget. You will be healthier, happier, and stronger.

If you decide that you do want to get even, remember the adage that says: "A good life is the best revenge." Then forgive and forget. Your happier life will be revenge enough.

Find things that make you laugh. It isn't too surprising that doing fun things can reduce our cortisol levels. It is surprising, however, to learn that even thinking about having fun can reduce our cortisol. Lee Berk and colleagues measured several hormone levels in eight young men, then told them that they were going to see a funny video in three days. Additional hormone measurements showed that stress hormone levels dropped at a progressively faster rate as the time for viewing the video approached.[2] By the time the video was being shown, cortisol levels had dropped 39 percent. Equally interesting was the fact that growth hormone levels climbed 87 percent. Growth hormone counteracts some of the effects of cortisol.

Live within your means. I couldn't find any research on the effects of living on the edge, scraping by from one paycheck to the next, staying up to watch one more program on TV every night, or eating on the run, but I think it's a safe bet that your hypothalamus doesn't like any of those things. Americans tend to live right on the edge of their physical, emotional, and financial limits, a characteristic that was observed more than a hundred years ago by Thomas Clouston, a Scottish psychiatrist:

> You Americans wear too much expression on your faces. You are living like an army with all its reserves engaged in action. The duller countenances of the British population betoken a better scheme of life. They suggest stores of reserved nervous force to fall back upon, if any occasion should arise that requires it. This inexcitability, this presence at all times of power not used, I regard as the great safeguard of our British people.[3]

The American habit of "burning the candle at both ends," has made the United States a wealthy and powerful nation, but the cost in stress-related illnesses is very high. As we get older we should slow down, relax, and try to accumulate reserves of Dr. Clouston's "nervous force."

Marry the right person. Marriage symbolizes a commitment to loving and being loved, two activities that reassure the hypothalamus that the world is a good and safe place. To expand our knowledge of relationships, Janice Kiecolt-Glaser and colleagues from Ohio State University measured the cortisol levels of ninety newlywed couples while they discussed their relationship history.[4] Later, the researchers counted the number of positive and negative terms each spouse had used in describing his or her marriage. Still later, the number of positive and negative terms used by the newlyweds was compared to changes in their cortisol levels.

The results of this experiment were complicated, but the finding of most interest here is that men and women who used positive terms to describe their marriage experienced a drop in their cortisol levels. This suggests that a good marriage lowers cortisol levels.

Get massages. Being touched seems to reassure the hypothalamus that the world is a good place. Getting massages lowered the cortisol levels of patients in the following categories: women with bulimia[5]; burn patients[6]; pregnant women[7]; and surgery patients.[8]

Trust God. Trusting that the Universe is in the hands of a benign spirit helps us cope with stressors. Gail Ironson and colleagues from the University of Miami in Florida conducted a study to find out whether spirituality, religiousness, or both were related to the long-term survival of people with AIDS.[9] They found that longer survival times were linked to a sense of peace; faith in God; religious behavior; and a compassionate view of others.

When the researchers analyzed their results to learn which characteristics linked spirituality and religiousness to the health of AIDS patients, they found two: altruism and low urinary cortisol levels. I think that Dr. Ironson and her colleagues have confirmed what all of the great religions teach—we will be healthier and happier if we mellow out, have faith, behave ourselves, and love one another.

MUSIC INCREASES STRESS RESISTANCE

The production of cortisol is controlled by the optimistic and musical right side of the brain, so it is probably not an accident that both optimism and music reduce cortisol production. Optimism and music also enhance immunity and recovery from illness. Here are a few research snippets showing the effects of music on various conditions.

Anxiety. Many patients are uneasy before surgery, so hospitals often have someone discuss the surgery with patients ahead of time. Unfortunately, the discussions themselves are stressful enough to cause 50 percent increases in cortisol levels. To see if music reduced the stress caused by presurgery briefings, researchers from Poland had some of their patients listen to an hour of music immediately after their briefings.[10] The cortisol levels of the patients who listened to music returned to normal within an hour. The patients who did not hear the music still had high cortisol levels an hour after their briefings ended.

Cancer. Cancer patients who attended a music program had lower cortisol levels afterward, and there were signs that their immune systems had been stimulated.[11]

Hypertension. Not all kinds of music are equally relaxing. Martin Möckel and colleagues, from the Free University in Berlin, Germany, examined twenty healthy young people before and after they listened to music selected by the researchers.[12] The three pieces of music—about six minutes long in each case—were parts of a waltz by Johann Strauss, a rondo by Hans Werner Henze, and a raga by Ravi Shankar. Cortisol levels dropped after each musical selection, but the only drop that was statistically significant was after the music of Ravi Shankar, as any hippie from the 1960s could have predicted.

A year later, Dr. Möckel and his associates repeated their musical experiment, but this time they included a group of patients with hypertension.[13] The patients with hypertension had higher cortisol levels than the healthy patients under all circumstances, but they still experienced a decrease in cortisol levels after listening to the music (Figure 19.1).

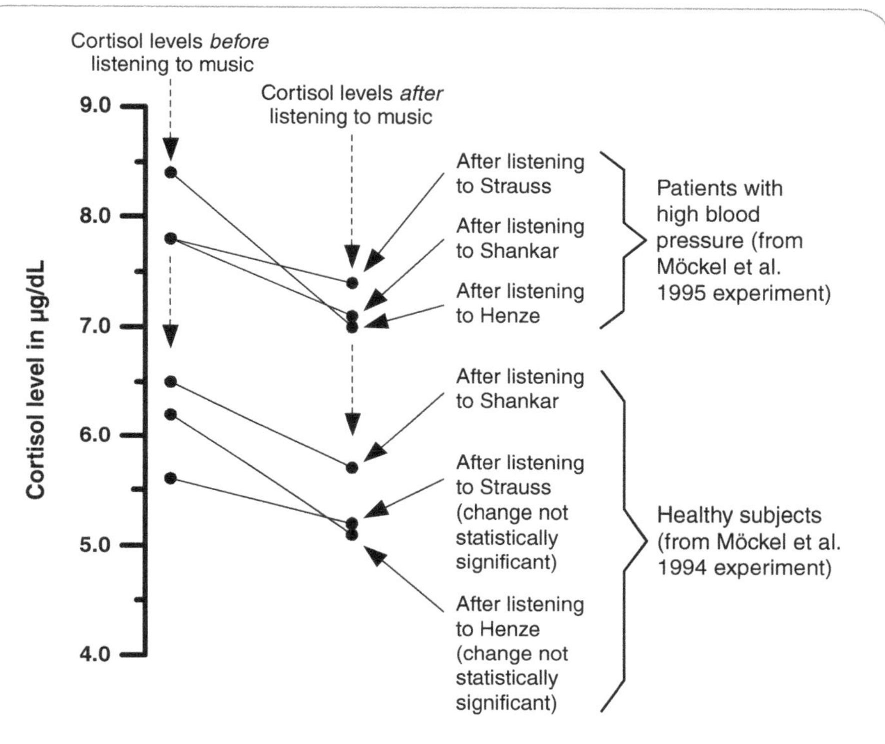

Figure 19.1. The Effects of Music on Cortisol Levels

Martin Möckel and colleagues presented three kinds of music to subjects with and without high blood pressure. All three types of music lowered the cortisol levels of both healthy and hypertensive subjects. Notice that the the hypertensive subjects had higher cortisol levels than the healthy subjects under all test conditions.

Mild discomfort. Researchers from the Hanover Medical School in Germany measured stress markers of patients undergoing mildly unpleasant examinations. Patients examined without music had elevated blood pressure and cortisol levels, but there was no change in the blood pressure and cortisol levels of patients who listened to music during their examinations.[14] The patients who had been the most fearful benefited the most from music.

REDUCING TENSION AND HYPERVIGILANCE

Two common reactions to stress are muscle tension and a narrowly focused alertness called *hypervigilance.* These conditions appear to be stress-induced stressors because they continue to stimulate cortisol production after the original stressor is gone. Several methods of reducing muscle tension and hypervigilance are described below.

Biofeedback. In biofeedback training, students use electronic devices to monitor body parameters such as muscle tension, blood pressure, or brain waves. The students are then taught to alter those parameters in ways that will be beneficial to them. For example, they may learn to reduce their muscle tension while watching an *electromyograph* (EMG) machine. Then they are taught to reduce their muscle tension *without* the electromyograph machine. A. V. McGrady, working with many other investigators, measured the effects of EMG training on blood pressure and other stress markers. Here are some of their findings:

- **Study 1**—Biofeedback trainees lowered their mean blood pressure from 144/90 to 133/84 mm Hg. Their cortisol levels dropped significantly during the study period.[15]
- **Study 2**—The trainees who benefited the most from an EMG biofeedback program were the ones with the highest levels of cortisol.[16]
- **Study 3**—When a group of people with normal blood pressure (normotensive) and a hypertensive group received identical biofeedback training, both groups significantly reduced their muscle tension. The cortisol levels and blood pressure of the normotensive group did not change, but the cortisol levels and blood pressure of the hypertensive group dropped.[17]
- **Study 4**—The hypertensive trainees who were most likely to benefit from biofeedback were those who had cool hands, high heart rates, high anxiety scores, and high cortisol levels.[18]
- **Study 5**—When successful trainees were examined a year later, they still had lower muscle tension, anxiety levels, and urinary cortisol than they had had before the training.[19]

The success of biofeedback in reducing blood pressure has prompted some HMOs to offer it to their clients, either free or at a very low price.

Cognitive behavioral stress management (CBSM). Chronic pain, stress, or illness can cause us to develop bad habits that lead to more pain, stress, and illness. CBSM tries to break this vicious cycle by teaching people how to relax, think more clearly, and improve their relationships with other people. Researchers from Florida studied a group of men with HIV who were taking a CBSM class. As expected, the subjects' cortisol levels dropped steadily as the course progressed.[20] Furthermore, the subjects who spent the most time doing the CBSM exercises had the largest reduction in their cortisol levels.

Emotional self-management. The Heartmath Institute teaches people how to manage their emotions. Researchers from the institute reported that people who took one of their short courses were able to reduce their cortisol levels by 23 percent.[21] Listening to music is part of Heartmath training.

Progressive relaxation training. When I was about ten, my friends and I would practice relaxing our muscles, starting with our toes and working up to our scalps. We didn't know it at the time, but we were practicing a technique called *progressive muscle relaxation.* This technique was developed in the 1930s to help people resist chronic illnesses.

My friends and I were not trying to resist illness; we were trying to get high. Progressively relaxing each muscle led to a very pleasant altered state of consciousness. With practice, it became possible to walk, swim, and ride our bikes in this relaxed but alert state. As I got older, and developed more bad habits, it became increasingly difficult to achieve this blissful state.

Laura Pawlow and Gary Jones recently published a report describing how progressive muscle relaxation reduced the heart rate, anxiety, feelings of stress, and cortisol levels of their subjects.[22]

Qi gong (or qigong). In some of the Eastern healing and martial arts, it is believed that a vital energy called *qi* flows through people, and the key to both health and mastery of the martial arts lies in controlling qi. Qi gong teaches people to control their qi through movement, meditation, and breathing exercises. A researcher from Hong Kong found that practicing qi gong, even for just a few weeks, reduced the cortisol levels of healthy subjects.[23]

Tai chi. Another word for *qi* is *chi,* and *tai chi* is a martial art that teaches control of *chi.* P. Jin, from La Trobe University in Bundoora, Australia, found that tai chi reduced the cortisol levels of practitioners. Furthermore, tai chi practitioners reported less anger, anxiety, confusion, depression, fatigue, and tension.[24] A few years later, Dr. Jin studied the stress-relieving qualities of tai chi, brisk walking, meditation, and neutral reading. Dr. Jin found that all four treatments reduced cortisol levels.[25]

Transcendental meditation (TM). Practitioners of transcendental meditation believe that repetition of a special sound called a *mantra* will help them to relax and focus their awareness. A 1978 study found that the cortisol levels of long-term practitioners decreased during meditation and remained somewhat low afterward.[26]

Yoga. "Alpha" waves from the brain are associated with relaxation, and the objective of many biofeedback techniques is to increase the amplitude of alpha waves. Researchers from Japan found that the alpha waves of yoga instructors increased, and cortisol levels decreased, while they were doing yoga exercises.[27] I studied both yoga and tai chi at various times, and I occasionally recaptured the same pleasant, peaceful state that I had experienced as a child practicing progressive muscle relaxation.

SLEEP IMPROVES STRESS RESISTANCE

Sleep, and especially deep, slow-wave sleep, boosts immunity and inhibits cortisol production.[28] Before electric light bulbs were invented, people spent a lot of time in bed because lighting a house with candles was expensive, dangerous, and dirty. As late as 1910, when electric lights were common, working people still slept about nine hours per night.[29] In 2002, Americans slept only 7.5 hours per night, and it is probably no accident that we are getting fatter as we stay awake longer. Chronic partial sleep deprivation causes a number of metabolic and endocrine changes, including:

- Increased cortisol secretion
- Decrease in growth hormone secretion
- Increased susceptibility to the dysmetabolic syndrome
- Alterations in glucose metabolism tending toward insulin resistance
- Increased sympathetic nervous activity
- Smaller nocturnal rise of thyrotropin (needed to stimulate thyroid gland)

The changes listed above are all accepted as normal parts of aging. But are they? Might we stay younger longer if we slept more? I think so.

EXERCISE KILLS GERMS

Moderate, enjoyable exercise increases our stress resistance by boosting immunity, reducing chronic pain, and counteracting depression. Conventional wisdom attributes the benefits of exercise to weight loss, but that is a poor explanation because very few people ever lose weight by exercising. A much better explanation can be derived from the fact that moderate, pleasant exercise kills germs.

The body has two overlapping circulatory systems. The cardiovascular system uses the heart to pump blood through all of our organs and tissues. Blood contains a fluid called lymph, and all of our cells are bathed in a slow-moving stream of lymph. The lymph flushes out germs, dead cells, and other detritus from between the cells. Lymph does not immediately return to the bloodstream—first, it has to be filtered by the lymphatic system.

Lymph is pumped through lymphatic vessels and filters by the contraction and relaxation of our muscles, so the amount of filtering done by the lymphatic system is proportional to the amount of exercise we get. We don't have to contract our muscles vigorously, but we have to contract and relax them often to make the filters work efficiently.

The filters in the lymphatic system are called *lymphoid organs* and they include the appendix, thymus, spleen, tonsils, and lymph nodes. These organs contain special cells for removing unwanted materials from the lymph, and they contain billions of immune cells. If we don't get enough exercise, these cells sit idle when they should be filtering lymph and killing germs.

If we exercise too much, we can raise our cortisol levels high enough to suppress the operation of the immune cells in the lymphoid organs. This will make us more susceptible to infections and reduce our resistance to stress.

EXERCISE REDUCES INFLAMMATION

Since moderate exercise kills germs, we would expect it to reduce inflammation, and it does. J. Kelly Smith and colleagues, from East Tennessee State University, studied the effects of supervised exercise on the inflammatory cytokines of forty-three subjects, all of whom were at high risk for heart attacks. The subjects exercised about two and a half hours a week for six months.[30] In addition to taking the usual measurements you would expect in a study of this kind, Smith and colleagues also measured the levels of the following cytokines:

"Bad" cytokines (atherogenic)	"Good" cytokines (atheroprotective)
IL-1 alpha	IL-4
TNF-alpha	IL-10
IFN gamma	TGF-beta 1

The "bad" cytokines are associated with infections, inflammation, and atherosclerosis. Bad cytokines IL-1 and TNF-alpha both stimulate cortisol production. The three "good" cytokines are anti-inflammatory.

By the end of the exercise program, the level of bad cytokines had fallen by 58 percent and the good cytokines had risen 36 percent. Levels of CRP, an important marker for inflammation, had dropped 35 percent. There was a dose-response relationship between the amount of time exercised and the changes in cytokines and CRP, meaning that those who exercised the most got the biggest benefit. Moderate, pleasant exercise feels good, builds muscles, strengthens our cardiopulmonary system, kills germs, and reduces inflammation. All of these actions increase our stress resistance.

SUPPLEMENTS CAN REPAIR DAMAGE DONE BY CPN INFECTIONS

Chlamydophila pneumoniae (CPN) infections damage cells, and the damaged cells produce inflammatory cytokines that stimulate cortisol production. Anything we can do to help our cells resist CPN infections should lower cortisol levels and boost our immunity.

Dr. David Wheldon, whose anti-CPN protocol was mentioned in Chapter 3, believes that we can reduce CPN-related cell damage by taking the following supplements daily:

- Acetyl-L-carnitine, 500 milligrams (Helps repair mitochondria damaged by CPN; mitochondria help convert food to energy.)
- Acidophilus capsules (Replaces friendly germs killed by antibiotics.)
- Alpha-lipoic acid, 150 milligrams (Helps repair mitochondria damaged by CPN.)
- Calcium, 500 milligrams
- Fish oil capsule (Repairs tissues damaged by infections.)
- Magnesium, 300 milligrams (Corrects low levels of magnesium found in patients with chronic infections.)
- Selenium, 100 micrograms (Repairs tissues damaged by CPN.)
- Vitamin B_{12}, 5,000 micrograms (Corrects low levels of B_{12} found in the cells of CPN patients.)
- Vitamin B complex, high dose (Repairs nerves damaged by CPN.)
- Vitamin C, 1,000 milligrams (Antioxidant; reduces free radical damage caused by CPN infections.)

- Vitamin D, 1,000 IU (Repairs endothelial cells damaged by CPN.)
- Vitamin E, 800 IU (Antioxidant; repairs connective tissues damaged by chronic infections.)

These supplements will not cure a CPN infection, but they will help you look and feel better. You can learn more about these and other supplements in the books recommended at the end of this chapter.

SUMMARY

The hypothalamus, which controls cortisol production, evolved to help cavemen deal with predators, famine, and acute infections. It is not very well adapted to help office workers cope with noise, traffic, and chronic infections. To stay healthy and happy in today's world, we need to continually reassure the hypothalamus that the world is a safe, kind, and beautiful place. We can convince the hypothalamus that everything is OK by convincing our higher brain centers that everything is OK. This is a difficult task, but it is one that experts have been studying since at least the time of Gautama Buddha, and there is a huge body of literature on how to feel safe, to love one another, and to see beauty in the world as it exists at this moment. Almost any church, mosque, synagogue, or temple on the planet can give you practical advice on the basic requirements for a happy, healthy life. The advice typically recommends trusting god, forgiving your enemies, and laughing a lot. As we saw above, all of these things lower cortisol levels.

Meditation, massage, qi gong, tai chi, yoga, relaxation training, and some kinds of music all stretch out the time between cortisol pulses. Mild exercise and some supplements can reduce inflammation and reduce cortisol production.

Anything that makes us healthier and calmer helps to build stress resistance. Stress resistance, in turn, helps us stay healthy and calm.

RECOMMENDED READING AND RESOURCES

All I Really Need to Know I Learned in Kindergarten, by Robert Fulghum (Ballantine Books, 2003).

This is a nice book. I wish I had read it before my heart attack.

The Alpha Lipoic Acid Breakthrough, by Burt Berkson, M.D. (Three Rivers Press, 1998).

Describes the many benefits of alpha-lipoic acid.

Anatomy of an Illness, by Norman Cousins (WW Norton, 1995).

In this famous book, Cousins tells how he recovered from a terrible illness by watching funny movies and taking lots of vitamin C.

Dr. Atkins' Vita-Nutrient Solution: Nature's Answer to Drugs, by Robert C. Atkins, M.D. (Fireside, 1999).

Dr Atkins became famous for his high-protein diet, but he was also an expert on vitamins and other supplements. This book is not only informative, it is a pleasure to read.

The Healing Factor: Vitamin C Against Disease, by Irwin Stone (Putnam, 1974).

In this 1972 book, Irwin Stone summarized years of work on the importance of vitamin C. Norman Cousins, Linus Pauling, and many others have written about the importance of this book, and I can't recommend it enough.

The HeartMath Solution, by Doc Lew Childre and Howard Martin (HarperSan-Francisco, 2000).

This book has many practical techniques designed to help us live happy, tranquil lives. The theories behind the techniques are a little strange, but no stranger than the theories behind yoga.

How to Age Rapidly or Not!, by Pauline N. Harding (NOHA News 2002 Winter; 27(1):3-6).

In this article, Dr. Harding gives a great deal of practical information on lowering cortisol levels. The article is available at www.nutrition4health.org/NOHAnews/NNW02 HardingAging.htm

Lights Out: Sleep, Sugar, and Survival, by T.S. Wiley and Bent Formby (Atria, 2000).

I mentioned earlier that I didn't agree with everything written in any of the books that I recommend. This warning goes triple for Lights Out, *even though it is one of the few books that discuss cortisol in depth. There are about ten pages-worth of extraordinarily interesting ideas sprinkled through this badly written book. You can read a review of it that covers the best parts by getting a copy of* The Felix Newsletter, *issue number 120. It is available for $2.00 from:*

Felix Letter
P. O. Box 7094
Berkeley, California 94707

PDR for Nutritional Supplements, by Sheldon Hendler and David Rorvik, editors (Thomson Healthcare, 2001).

This is "the bible" for nutritional supplements. It is expensive and somewhat technical, but if you have chronic illnesses it would be worth a trip to the library to take a look at this book.

Prescription for Nutritional Healing, by Phyllis Balch and James Balch (Avery/Penguin Putnam, 2000).

An excellent book on vitamins, minerals, herbs, and nutritional supplements.

REFERENCES

Epigraph: National Institutes of Health. 2003. NIH Document RFA 08-03-004.

1. The Office of News and Public Affairs Stanford University Medical Center. Women who need to forgive someone sought for participation in Stanford study of health effects of anger. News release, May 22, 2001.

2. Berk, Lee et al. Expecting a laugh boosts stress-busting hormones. Paper presented at the 2002 Society for Neuroscience meeting in Orlando, FL, described in a press release from the University of Califonia, at Irvine. November 6, 2002. http://today.uci.edu/news/release_detail.asp?key=942.

3. Clouston, Thomas, quoted by William James. "The Gospel of Relaxation." www.emory.edu/EDUCATION/mfp/jgospel.html.

4. Positive Encounters Lowered Stress Reactions and Influenced Longevity of Relationship, Especially for Wives. APA News Release, August 2000.

5. Field T, Schanberg S, Kuhn C, et al. Bulimic adolescents benefit from massage therapy. *Adolescence* 1998 Fall;33(131):555–563.

6. Field T, Peck M, Krugman S, et al. Burn injuries benefit from massage therapy. *J Burn Care Rehabil* 1998 May-Jun;19(3):241–244.

7. *The Osgood File: Maternal Massage.* CBS Radio Network, 2001 Feb. KRON-TV San Francisco.

8. Kim MS, Cho KS, Woo H, et al. Effects of hand massage on anxiety in cataract surgery using local anesthesia. *J Cataract Refract Surg* 2001 Jun;27(6):884–890.

9. Ironson G, Solomon GF, Balbin EG, et al. The Ironson-woods Spirituality/Religiousness Index is associated with long survival, health behaviors, less distress, and low cortisol in people with HIV/AIDS. *Ann Behav Med* 2002 Winter;24(1): 34–48.

10. Miluk-Kolasa B, Obminski Z, Stupnicki et al. Effects of music treatment on salivary cortisol in patients exposed to pre-surgical stress. *Exp Clin Endocrinol* 1994;102(2):118–120.

11. Burns SJ, Harbuz MS, Hucklebridge F, et al. A pilot study into the therapeutic effects of music therapy at a cancer help center. *Altern Ther Health Med* 2001 Jan;7(1):48–56.

12. Möckel M, Rocker L, Stork T, et al. Immediate physiological responses of healthy volunteers to different types of music: Cardiovascular, hormonal and mental changes. *Eur J Appl Physiol Occup Physiol* 1994;68(6):451–459.

13. Möckel M, Stork T, Vollert J, et al. [Stress reduction through listening to music: effects on stress hormones, hemodynamics and mental state in patients with arterial hypertension and in healthy persons [Article in German]. *Dtsch Med Wochenschr* 1995 May 26;120(21):745–752.

14. Schneider N, Schedlowski M, Schurmeyer TH, et al. Stress reduction through music in patients undergoing cerebral angiography. *Neuroradiology* 2001 Jun;43(6):472–476

15. McGrady AV, Yonker R, Tan SY, et al. The effect of biofeedback-assisted relaxation training on blood pressure and selected biochemical parameters in patients with essential hypertension. *Biofeedback Self Regul* 1981 Sep;6(3):343–353.

16. McGrady A, Utz SW, Woerner M, et al. Predictors of success in hypertensives treated with biofeedback-assisted relaxation. *Biofeedback Self Regul* 1986 Jun;11(2):95–103.

17. McGrady A, Woerner M, Bernal GA, et al. Effect of biofeedback-assisted relaxation on blood pressure and cortisol levels in normotensives and hypertensives. *J Behav Med* 1987 Jun;10(3):301–310.

18. McGrady A and Higgins JT Jr. Prediction of response to biofeedback-assisted relaxation in hypertensives: Development of a Hypertensive Predictor Profile (HYPP). *Psychosom Med* 1989 May-Jun;51(3):277–284.

19. McGrady A, Nadsady PA, and Schumann-Brzezinski C. Sustained effects of biofeedback-assisted relaxation therapy in essential hypertension. *Biofeedback Self Regul* 1991 Dec;16(4):399–411.

20. Cruess DG, Antoni MH, Kumar M, et al. Reductions in salivary cortisol are associated with mood improvement during relaxation training among HIV-seropositive men. *J Behav Med* 2000 Apr;23(2):107–122.

21. McCraty, R Barrios-Choplin B, Rozman D, et al. The Impact of a New Emotional Self-Management Program on Stress, Emotions, Heart Rate Variability, DHEA and Cortisol. *Integrative Physiological and Behavioral Science*, 1998; 33(2):151–170.

22. Pawlow LA and Jones GE. The impact of abbreviated progressive muscle relaxation on salivary cortisol. *Biol Psychol* 2002;60(1):1–16.

23. Jones BM. Changes in cytokine production in healthy subjects practicing Guolin Qigong : a pilot study. *BMC Complement Altern Med* 2001;1(1):8.

24. Jin P. Changes in heart rate, noradrenaline, cortisol and mood during Tai Chi. *J Psychosom Res* 1989;33(2):197–206.

25. Jin P. Efficacy of Tai Chi, brisk walking, meditation, and reading in reducing mental and emotional stress. *J Psychosom Res* 1992 May;36(4):361–370.

26. Jevning R, Wilson AF, and Davidson JM. Adrenocortical activity during meditation. *Horm Behav* 1978 Feb;10(1):54–60.

27. Kamei T, Toriumi Y, Kimura H, et al. Decrease in serum cortisol during yoga exercise is correlated with alpha wave activation. *Percept Mot Skills* 2000 Jun;90(3 Pt 1):1027–1032.

28. Bierwolf C, Struve K, Marshall L, et al. Slow wave sleep drives inhibition of pituitary-adrenal secretion in humans. *J Neuroendocrinol* 1997 Jun;9(6):479–484.

29. National Institutes of Health. 2002 Oct. *Role of Sleep and Sleep-Disordered Breathing in Metabolic Syndrome.* RFA-HL-03-008.

30. Smith JK, Dykes R, Douglas JE, et al. Long-term exercise and atherogenic activity of blood mononuclear cells in persons at risk of developing ischemic heart disease. *JAMA* 1999 May 12;281(18):1722–1727.

20

Reversing Infection-Cortisol (IC) Loops

. . . . most cases of so-called "spontaneous remission" are not considered spontaneous at all by the person who actually recovers. . . . The person may attribute his or her recovery to a significant change in their life situation, a change in diet, a change in attitudes, adoption of a particular unconventional healing approach, or through spiritual/religious means such as prayer, faith, and divine intervention. In fact, those who have studied the phenomenon of spontaneous remission report that in most cases the person made a significant change from their previous ways of thinking, behaving, and living.

—RICHARD W. HANSON, PH.D., VETERANS ADMINISTRATION

Many cases of "spontaneous" remission appear to be examples of people reversing their infection-cortisol loops by avoiding stress or increasing their stress resistance. Sometimes these techniques produce results that can only be described as miraculous, but we cannot depend on them for two reasons. First, some germs are just too hard to kill, and no amount of stress reduction will eradicate them. Second, stress reduction requires us to change our behavior, and therapies that depend on behavior changes are notoriously ineffective. In this closing chapter, I want to propose an infection-cortisol reduction (ICR) program that encourages, but does not depend upon, behavioral changes. The program is based on research discussed in earlier chapters, so most of it will be familiar.

ONE LAST THOUGHT EXPERIMENT

When we left Clem at the end of the dieting thought experiment, he was in an awful fix, and things didn't get any better as he got older. We meet him again as he is being wheeled into an emergency room with wires on his chest and tubes in his nose. He's sixty, grossly overweight, depressed, and hypertensive. He has a dozen things wrong with him, but the problem that is getting attention now is a pain in his chest that runs through his left shoulder and down his arm.

The next day, Clem's doctor tells him he's had a mild heart attack. He doesn't need a bypass operation yet, but he will need one within a few years. He's discharged from the hospital and goes home feeling a hundred years old. While he is recuperating, a computer in the main office of his health insurance company calculates how much money the company is likely to spend on Clem during his remaining years. The computer concludes that the company might be able to save tens of thousands of dollars by paying for Clem to enroll in an infection-cortisol reduction (ICR) program. The computer promptly sends a form letter to Clem.

After Clem reads the letter, he makes a few phone calls, and two weeks later he checks into an ICR clinic for an overnight physical exam. In addition to the usual poking and prodding, the ICR team conducts the tests recommended by Dr. Mårin in Chapter 16. They also measure and check:

- Clem's cortisol levels at 8:00 A.M., 4:00 P.M., and midnight.
- His antibodies against twenty common germs.
- Prevalence of *Chlamydophila pneumoniae* (CPN) organisms in Clem's monocytes.
- His inflammatory cytokines: IL-1, IL-6, and TNF-alpha.
- His acute phase proteins, especially C-reactive protein (CRP).
- How well he sleeps.

A week later Clem returns to the clinic, and one of the ICR doctors explains the results of his tests. Clem has chronic subtle hypercortisolism (potbelly syndrome). His liver, kidneys, eyes, arteries, joints, nerves, and skeletal muscles have all been damaged by chronic infections, inflammation, hypertension, and insulin resistance.

The ICR doctor explains to Clem that he is infected with seven of the twenty germs he was tested for, but he will only be treated for one of them—CPN—at this time. Clem leaves the clinic with a reading list, a schedule of classes, a month's supply of supplements and medications, and an appointment to return to the clinic in four weeks. Clem's medications include antibiotics selected to kill both the active and the spore-like forms of CPN.

Clem takes his pills, reads the recommended books, and attends "Life 101" classes. He learns about his immune system, how cortisol is regulated, and how infections block our arteries. He studies meditation, yoga, biofeedback, and nutrition. He listens to carefully selected music before he goes to bed.

During the first month, Clem's cortisol level drops a little and he becomes less insulin resistant. Cells throughout his body begin to repair themselves. As the cellular repair goes on, he begins to feel better. When he returns to the clinic, blood tests show that his IL-1, IL-6, TNF-alpha, CRP, and antibody levels are all lower. He is still infected with CPN, however, so he is given another month's supply of medicine and supplements.

During his second month in the ICR program, Clem's infection-cortisol loop reverses itself and becomes an immunity-health loop. He gets healthier every day. His potbelly is shrinking and his blood pressure is dropping. As his joints and muscles repair themselves, Clem rediscovers the simple joys of moving, and he finds himself taking long walks just for the pleasure of feeling his legs move.

Clem looks better and feels great, but PCR tests show that his monocytes are still infected with CPN. This is a critical point in Clem's treatment—he is very happy with the results of the program, but quitting now would be disastrous.

Let's imagine that Clem has only one viable CPN organism left in his body. This last organism—we can call it "Spud" since CPN organisms look like potatoes—is fine-tuned to live in Clem's body. Spud's ancestors outwitted Clem's immune system for roughly 15,000 generations, and Spud is the toughest, meanest, wiliest CPN organism that selective breeding can produce. If Clem drops out of the ICR program before Spud dies, then Spud will reproduce, and Spud's offspring will be far nastier than his ancestors were. Spud's ancestors needed thirty years to wreck Clem's health, but Spud's descendents will only need a few months.

The point of the Spud story is that it is not enough to treat an infection until the patient feels better—middle-path infections should be treated until the target germ is eradicated, either by drugs, or by the patient's immune system. When the immune system is working at its best, it can kill germs that drugs can't touch.

Fortunately, Clem stays in our hypothetical ICR program until Spud is dead. With his monocytes free from infection, and his cortisol level reduced,

Clem's immune system is in tip-top shape and it eradicates some of his other infections without any help from the ICR team. With lower cortisol levels and no CPN infection, Clem's macrophages begin to remove excess cholesterol from his arteries.

YOU MAY BE ABLE TO START YOUR OWN ICR PROGRAM

The ICR program described above is not very far-fetched. There are laboratories in every large city that can do the necessary tests. The antibiotics required are in common use and reasonably safe. Every community college offers courses like those that Clem took.

If you are not bound by the rules of HMOs and insurance companies, you can start a one-person ICR program for yourself. The biggest hurdle will be to find a doctor, or a combination of doctors, who understand both infections and cortisol.

If you do start your own ICR program, and find that you are infected with CPN, give your doctors copies of the antichlamydial protocols discussed in Chapter 3. Make sure that your ICR team doesn't stop treating you until your last CPN organism is dead. In my own case, I had a brief but spectacular improvement in my health following my first clarithromycin treatment. Since no attempt was made to eradicate my last CPN organism, I became ill again within a few months. I believe that most of my subsequent illnesses could have been prevented if my HMO doctors had followed the protocol sent to them by Dr. Stratton.

If you work for an insurance company, and you are wondering whether an ICR program would save money for your company, consider running a pilot study. Any HMO or university hospital could conduct such a study for the cost of a few triple-bypass operations.

USING ANTICORTISOL DRUGS TO REVERSE IC LOOPS

It may be possible to reverse IC loops by forcing cortisol levels down with drugs. This would allow the immune system to kill more germs. Unfortunately, forcing our cortisol levels down will impair our ability to cope with inflammation and other stressors. It seems better, when possible, to reduce stress rather than block cortisol production. It may be necessary to use anticortisol drugs to treat people who produce too much cortisol even when they are unstressed and have few infections. One of the most powerful of these drugs is an antifungal medicine called ketoconazole. It inhibits or blocks the production of all steroids, including cortisol, and it is sometimes used to treat patients with Cushing's syndrome. Dr. Mårin is studying a derivative of ketoconazole to see if it can be developed into a safe treatment for PBS. Early results have been good, but more study is needed.

The anticortisol drugs I have studied are so dangerous, and their use is so complicated, that they should only be used under the supervision of specially trained physicians, usually endocrinologists.

SUMMARY

When Pandora opened her famous box, all of the evils and illnesses that had been trapped in it escaped and spread throughout the world. Like Pandora's box, an IC loop produces a steady stream of illnesses including heart disease, obesity, hypertension, and type 2 diabetes. This stream can be slowed down, and sometimes reversed, by reducing cortisol levels or eradicating infections. Cortisol levels can be reduced by changing our behavior, but the results are uncertain. Some infections can be eradicated, but middle-path germs such as CPN are particularly hard to kill.

We now know enough about detecting and killing CPN organisms that an ICR program could be started with a reasonable chance of success in those cases where CPN is a major source of inflammation. As our knowledge grows, ICR programs could be extended to combat other germs.

Conclusion

Before my heart attack, I believed that heart disease and potbellies were caused by too much food and not enough exercise. I was wrong. In *The Potbelly Syndrome,* Dr. Mårin and I have shown how these problems, and many others, are actually caused by stress and chronic infections. More specifically, we have shown how:

- Common germs, not hamburgers, cause heart disease.
- Germs increase our stress levels.
- Stress causes chronic subtle hypercortisolism (potbelly syndrome).
- Chronic subtle hypercortisolism causes insulin resistance, potbellies, high blood pressure, and type 2 diabetes.
- We can improve our chances of having "spontaneous" remissions.
- Calorie-restriction diets make us gain weight.

Some foods are clearly better for us than others, but no change in the kind or amount of food we eat will ever eradicate the germs that cause heart disease. Similarly, moderate exercise is good for us, but it can't eliminate the stress caused by chronic infections. If we want to have healthy hearts and flat stomachs, we need to:

- Reduce our exposure to stress (Chapter 18).
- Increase our resistance to stress (Chapter 19).
- Eradicate our chronic infections (Chapter 20).

You can lower your stress levels by yourself, but you will need the help of a pretty sharp doctor to eradicate your chronic infections. Don't be surprised if your family doctor drags her feet when you ask to be tested for *Chlamydophila pneumoniae* or hypercortisolism. The ideas presented here are new, and new ideas mean more work for your doctor. Be patient. On the other hand, if you can't wait months or years for her to order the tests you need, read Chapter 17 again. Don't give up.

Glossary

Abdominal sagittal diameter (ASD). The distance from the back to the highest part of the abdomen of a person lying on his or her back. It should be less than ten inches.

Acquired immunodeficiency syndrome (AIDS). A syndrome characterized by high cortisol levels and a breakdown of the body's immune defenses. It is caused by the human immunodeficiency virus (HIV).

Acute phase proteins (APPs). Proteins produced by the liver during an acute phase response. The best known of these is C-reactive protein (CRP), a marker for inflammation.

Acute phase response (APR). The body's response to injury or infection. APRs produce inflammatory substances to kill germs, and then produce anti-inflammatory substances to protect the body from the inflammatory ones. (Sometimes called *acute phase reaction*.)

Adenovirus. A common virus widely used in experiments in which genes are inserted into human cells. It causes obesity in animals.

Adrenal glands. Glands that produce many hormones, including cortisol, aldosterone, epinephrine, and norepinephine.

Adrenocorticotropic hormone (ACTH). A hormone produced by the pituitary gland that stimulates the production of cortisol.

Afternoon cortisol level. Cortisol level measured eight hours after a morning cortisol measurement. It should be should be less than half of the morning level.

Aneurysm. A balloon-like bulge in an artery.

Angiopathy. A disease of the blood vessels. Macroangiopathy is a disease of the large vessels; microangiopathy is a disease of the small vessels.

Antibiotic. A medicine that kills bacteria.

Antibodies. Proteins that the body makes to kill germs. Also called *immunoglobulins.*

Anticortisol. A substance that resists the production or activity of cortisol.

Anti-inflammatory. Something that reduces inflammation.

Antistressors. Love, trust, laughter, and other things that reduce or neutralize the effects of stressors.

Aorta. The largest artery in the body.

Appestat. The systems that control hunger.

Appetite set point weight. Usually just called the "appetite set point." It is the weight at which you will stop gaining or losing weight if you eat whatever you wish without regard to health or appearance. Leptin lowers the appetite set point and cortisol raises it.

Artery. A blood vessel that carries blood away from the heart to other parts of the body.

Atheroma. A sore (lesion) filled with pus. This term is often used when describing sores in arteries.

Atherosclerosis. A disease of the arteries in which cholesterol-containing foam cells crawl into the walls of our arteries and die. The dead foam cells form streaks and cores of pus (atheromas) in the arteries. As the process continues, the arteries to the heart may narrow, cutting down the flow of blood and nutrients to the heart.

Atrial fibrillation. A condition in which the upper chambers of the heart beat faster than the lower chambers.

Bacterium. A single-celled germ. Many bacteria cause disease.

Biofeedback. The use of electronic devices to monitor body activities. Biofeedback techniques are used widely to teach relaxation and stress reduction.

Blood pressure. The force of the blood on the walls of arteries. Two levels of blood pressure are measured; systolic and diastolic. In a blood pressure reading of 120/80 (spoken as "120 over 80"), 120 is the systolic pressure and 80 is the diastolic pressure.

Body mass index (BMI). The BMI formula is weight in kilograms divided by height in meters squared. (BMI = kg/m^2).

Caffeine. An insect poison produced by coffee, tea, and other plants.

Calorie. Unit of measurement for energy. Carbohydrates and protein produce about four calories per gram when burned, while fat yields about nine calories per gram.

Capillaries. The smallest blood vessels. Capillary walls are so thin that oxygen, glucose, cytokines, and hormones can pass through them and enter our cells.

Carbohydrate. Sugars, starches, and fiber. The body can convert carbohydrates and protein—but not fat—to a sugar (glucose) and a starch (glycogen).

Cardiopulmonary system. The heart and lungs.

Cardiovascular disease (CVD). Disease of the heart or blood vessels. The most common form of CVD is atherosclerosis.

Cardiovascular system. The heart and blood vessels (arteries, veins, and capillaries). Also called the *circulatory system.*

Carotid arteries. Arteries that carry blood up through the neck to the brain.

Cataract. Clouding of the lens of the eye. Cataracts can be caused by excess cortisol.

Chlamydia pneumoniae. *See Chlamydophila pneumoniae* (CPN).

Chlamydia trachomatis. A sexually transmitted bacterium typically found in the eyes and/or the genitals. Worldwide, *C. trachomatis* is the most common cause of blindness.

***Chlamydophila pneumoniae* (CPN).** A bacterium that causes damage to lungs, arteries, and nerves. Also called *Chlamydia pneumoniae, Chlamydia* TWAR, or TWAR.

Cholesterol. A soft, waxy substance that is an important component of all cell membranes. Cholesterol is vital to the proper growth and functioning of the nervous system, muscles, skin, liver, intestines, and heart. The body uses cholesterol to make hormones, bile acid, and vitamin D.

Clarithromycin. An antibiotic used to kill bacteria such as *Chlamydophila pneumoniae.*

Computed tomography (CT). A diagnostic imaging procedure that produces cross-sectional images of body tissues and structures.

Coronary heart disease (CHD). Disease of the arteries supplying blood to the heart; most commonly atherosclerosis. Also called *coronary artery disease* or simply *heart disease.*

Corticotropin-releasing hormone (CRH). A hormone released by the hypothalamus when the total of background and transient stressors exceeds a threshold level in the body. CRH is sometimes called *corticotropin-releasing factor* (CRF).

Cortisol. A hormone that is produced by the outer layers (cortices) of the adrenal glands. It is important in the regulation of blood pressure, blood sugar, and immunity. Cortisol is normally released in sixteen to twenty pulses per day of about 1 milligram each.

Cortisol receptors. Areas on the outer part of a cell that allow the cell to bind with cortisol from the blood. *See also* Receptor.

Cortisol sensitivity. The degree to which the body responds to a given amount of cortisol.

Cortisol-release threshold. The total amount of background and transient stress required to trigger the release of a pulse of cortisol.

Cortisone. A glucocorticoid hormone that is chemically similar to cortisol. It is not as powerful, however.

C-reactive protein (CRP). An acute phase protein. CRP is an excellent marker for inflammation and infections.

Cushing's syndrome (CS). A disease caused by very high cortisol levels. CS closely resembles potbelly syndrome.

Cytokines. Proteins that cells use to "talk" to each other. Some cytokines promote inflammation and others reduce inflammation.

Cytokine cascade. The rapid increase in cytokines that occurs shortly after an infection begins. Part of an acute phase response.

Cytokine storm. A cytokine cascade that gets out of control. It can inflame every cell in the body in a few days. Cortisol normally prevents cytokine cascades from turning into cytokine storms.

Cytomegalovirus (CMV). One of the most common of the human herpes viruses. Also known as human herpes virus 5 (HHV-5).

Depression. A mental state marked in part by sadness, inactivity, difficulty concentrating, and feelings of hopelessness; commonly seen in people with hypercortisolism.

Dexamethasone (DEX). A cortisol-like medicine that suppresses cortisol production.

Dexamethasone test. A test to see how well the HPA axis can regulate cortisol levels.

Diabetes. A disease in which the body is unable to properly process and use blood sugar (glucose). Often called diabetes mellitus.

Diabetes, gestational. Diabetes that occurs during pregnancy.

Diabetes, steroid-induced. A type of diabetes caused by cortisol-like medicines. It is similar to type 2 diabetes.

Diabetes, type 1. A type of diabetes in which the pancreas makes little or no insulin because the insulin-producing beta cells have been destroyed. This disease is also called *insulin-dependent diabetes mellitus* (IDDM).

Diabetes, type 2. A type of diabetes in which the pancreas makes insulin, but it is ineffective because of insulin resistance. It is often called *noninsulin-dependent diabetes mellitus* (NIDDM).

Diastolic blood pressure. The blood pressure that exists when the heart rests between beats.

Diurnal cycle. The daily rise and fall of the level of a substance in the body.

Diurnal cycle, flattened. Daily cycle of a substance in the body that does not have the normal peaks or valleys.

Dyslipidemia. Improper levels of fats and cholesterol in the blood.

Dysmetabolic syndrome X (DSX). This is currently (2005) the name used by the NIH for its expanded version of Reaven's syndrome X. This term will probably be replaced by *insulin resistance syndrome.*

Dysmetabolic syndromes. Any of the dozens of expanded versions of Reaven's syndrome X (RSX). Like RSX, all of the dysmetabolic syndromes have insulin resistance as their central feature, and most of them include high LDL cholesterol, low HDL cholesterol, and high blood pressure. Unlike RSX, most of the dysmetabolic syndromes include abdominal/visceral obesity.

Dysphoria. An unpleasant feeling. The opposite of euphoria.

Endocrine glands. Glands that secrete hormones into the bloodstream. For example, the adrenal glands secrete cortisol, aldosterone, epinephrine, norepinephine, and other hormones. The pancreas secretes insulin.

Endogenous. Grown or made inside the body.

Endothelial cells. Delicate cells lining the insides of organs and arteries that control the flow of nutrients and hormones to other cells.

Endotoxin. A poison contained in the cell walls of bacteria; it is released into our blood when a bacterium dies.

Epidemiology. The study of who has what diseases.

Epigastric pains. Stomach pains.

Euphoria. A pleasant or elated feeling; sometimes a side effect of cortisol-like medicines.

Eustress. Stress that is positive and healthy, such as that from walking your grandkids down to the corner to buy them ice cream.

Exogenous. Produced outside of the body.

Fat cells. Cells that convert glucose and fatty acids to triglycerides (fat) for long-term storage. When food is scarce, fat cells release fatty acids and glycerol into the blood for fuel.

Fat, abdominal. Fat around and in the abdomen; includes subcutaneous and visceral fat.

Fat, subcutaneous. Fat under the skin.

Fat, visceral. Fat surrounding the inner organs.

Fats. Efficient substances for storing energy. Fat is stored in the form of triglycerides.

Fats, saturated. Fats that are solid at room temperature. Examples include butter, lard, meat fat, solid shortening, palm oil, and coconut oil. The body uses saturated fats to make cholesterol when needed.

Fats, unsaturated. Fats that are liquid at room temperature. Examples include oils from olives, peanuts, corn, cottonseeds, sunflower seeds, safflower seeds, and soybeans. The body does not use these fats to produce cholesterol. Some of these fats are highly inflammatory and suppress the immune system.

Fat-storage set point (FSSP) weight. The weight at which we burn fuel at the same rate we are taking it in.

Fatty acids. Fat molecules.

Fatty liver. *See* Steatosis.

Feedback loop. In a control system, part of the output may be returned to the input to regulate the output.

Foam cells. Cells other than fat cells that contain large quantities of fat. The foam cells of greatest interest in this book are diseased macrophages that fill up with cholesterol and then die in arteries, thus causing atherosclerosis.

Germ. Any bacterium, virus, or other microorganism.

Glucocorticoids. A group of anti-inflammatory hormones that affect carbohydrate metabolism. They also play a role in fat and protein metabolism, maintenance of blood pressure, and the functioning of the central nervous system. Cortisol is the most important glucocorticoid.

Glucose (blood sugar). The simplest form of sugar. The body normally makes glucose from carbohydrates, but it can also make glucose from proteins when carbohydrates are scarce. Glucose is the main source of energy for living cells, but some cells cannot use it without the help of insulin.

Glucose intolerance. The inability of the body to maintain an optimal glucose level after consuming carbohydrates. This condition often precedes diabetes.

Glucose tolerance test. A test given to see how well the body deals with a surge of glucose.

Glycogen. The stored form of glucose found in the liver and muscles. The body can only store enough glycogen to fuel the body for a few hours, and then it must begin to metabolize proteins or triglycerides for fuel.

Heart attack. An interruption of blood flow to the heart that is severe enough to cause death to part of the heart muscle. Also called a *myocardial infarction* (MI) or an *acute myocardial infarction* (AMI).

Heart disease. Usually refers to coronary heart disease. *See* Coronary heart disease (CHD).

Helicobacter pylori (H. pylori). A bacterium that causes peptic ulcers and stomach cancer. It may also cause weight gain or loss depending upon other health factors. It is suspected of causing atherosclerosis in some people and is associated with diabetes and obesity.

Hemoglobin A1c (HbA1c). A substance in the body, levels of which indicate the severity of a person's diabetes.

Herpes simplex viruses (HSV1 and HSV2). Middle-path germs that have been implicated in causing atherosclerosis. They are two of the eight known human herpes viruses.

High blood pressure. Greater than normal force pushing against arterial walls. High blood pressure strains the heart; harms the arteries; and increases the risk of heart attack, stroke, and kidney problems. Also called *hypertension.*

Hormones. Chemicals secreted by some cells to tell other cells what to do.

HPA axis. Hypothalamic-pituitary-adrenal axis. The adrenal glands produce and regulate cortisol. The hypothalamus and the pituitary gland regulate how much cortisol is produced.

Human growth hormone (HGH). A hormone with some anticortisol qualities. Often called *growth hormone* (*GH*).

Hypercortisolism. Too much cortisol in the blood. Sometimes called *hypercortisolemia.*

Hyperglycemia. Too much glucose in the blood.

Hyperinsulinism. Too much insulin in the blood; a frequent marker for dysmetabolic syndromes. Also called *hyperinsulinemia.*

Hyperlipidemia. High levels of fats (lipids) in the blood; a symptom of hypercortisolism.

Hyperplasia. Abnormal proliferation of cells.

Hypertension. Excessive force pressing against arterial walls; also called *high blood pressure.*

Hypertension, primary. The most common form of hypertension. Also called *essential hypertension.*

Hypertrophy. Excessive growth.

Hypocortisolism. Low cortisol levels. Extreme hypocortisolism is called *Addison's disease.*

Hypoglycemia. Too little glucose in the blood.

Hypotension. Low blood pressure or a sudden drop in blood pressure.

Hypothalamic-pituitary-adrenal axis. *See* HPA axis.

Hypothalamus. The part of the brain that regulates cortisol and thyroid levels.

Hypoxia. Not enough oxygen in the blood; stimulates cortisol production.

Iatrogenic. Refers to health problems caused by medical treatments.

Immune system. The cells and organs that defend the body against infection and cancer.

Impaired glucose tolerance (IGT). Glucose levels higher than normal but not high enough to be called diabetes.

Incidentaloma. A tumor on the adrenal gland usually discovered by accident during medical procedures.

Infection. Invasion of a host by a germ, with the subsequent multiplication and establishment of the germ. An infection may or may not lead to disease.

Inflammation. Redness, warmth, swelling, pain, and loss of function produced in response to infection. It is the result of an influx of immune cells and cytokines, plus increased blood flow, into the inflamed tissues.

Inflammatory cytokines. Cytokines that tend to increase inflammation. The primary cytokines IL-1, IL-6, and TNF-alpha are inflammatory. *See* Cytokines.

Insulin. A hormone that helps to move glucose out of the blood and into liver, muscle, and fat cells. It is produced by the pancreas.

Insulin resistance. The inability of liver and muscle cells to respond to insulin. This prevents cells from using glucose effectively. Insulin resistance is the central defect in all of the dysmetabolic syndromes, including potbelly syndrome.

Insulin resistance syndrome. This term is gradually replacing the other terms used for the various dysmetabolic syndromes.

Insulin-dependent diabetes mellitus (IDDM). *See* Diabetes, type 1.

Interleukin-1 (IL-1). Inflammatory cytokine, one of the primary cytokines that raise cortisol levels.

Interleukin-6 (IL-6). Inflammatory cytokine, one of the primary cytokines that raise cortisol levels.

Intima. *See* Tunica intima.

Intracellular germs. Germs that live and reproduce inside of cells. Generally, the immune system can only kill intracellular germs by killing the cells in which they live. Some antibiotics can kill intracellular germs without killing the cells.

Ischemia, myocardial. Insufficient blood supply to the heart muscle caused by a decreased capacity of the coronary vessels.

Ischemic heart disease (IHD). Ischemic (blocked-artery) heart disease.

Ju Ju. West African term for magic. Can be good or bad.

Kidneys. Two organs in the lower back that act as filters to remove wastes and poisons from the blood. The kidneys convert a substantial amount of cortisol to a less active hormone called cortisone. The kidneys are important in the regulation of blood pressure, and they are easily damaged by high blood pressure. Kidney disease is called *nephropathy.*

Kwashiorkor. Severe deficiency of proteins. Children with kwashiorkor often have tiny limbs and large potbellies. They also have extremely high cortisol levels. Compare with marasmus.

Leptin. A hormone produced by fat cells. Leptin levels tell the appestat and lipostat how much fat we are storing. Leptin may be an important stress hormone, and it appears to protect us from severe infections.

Leptin resistance. A condition in which the hypothalamus does not respond properly to leptin.

Lesion. An injury or sore.

Lipids. Fats, including cholesterol and triglycerides.

Lipostat. The systems that regulate fat storage. Lipostats were called *ponderostats* for many years, and they are sometimes called *adipostats* now.

Liver. A large organ that helps to regulate blood sugar levels. It produces acute phase proteins (APPs) to help us survive infections and inflammations.

Macrophages. Very large white blood cells that begin life as monocytes. They are often infected with *Chlamydophila pneumoniae*. Diseased macrophages fill up with cholesterol and become foam cells.

Malaise. A feeling of general discomfort or uneasiness. Often the first indication of an infection or other disease.

Marasmus. Severe deficiency of food of any kind. Children with marasmus have extremely high cortisol levels.

Marginally supraoptimal glucocorticoid activity. A carefully chosen phrase describing the cause of most cases of the potbelly syndrome.

Media. *See* tunica media.

Metabolic syndrome X. One of the many names given to versions of the dysmetabolic syndrome.

Metabolism. Chemical processes that occur within a living cell or organism. Metabolism includes breaking down substances to produce energy (catabolism) and synthesizing other substances (anabolism). Cortisol accelerates catabolic processes.

Middle-path germs. Germs that can survive in us for many years despite our best efforts to eradicate them. Infections caused by these germs flood the body with cortisol and other dangerous chemicals. Some species of middle-path germs, such as CMV and CPN, are often found together.

Midnight cortisol test. A measurement of blood cortisol level taken at midnight. This is a relatively new test, and it is a very important one for people who may have hypercortisolism.

Monocytes. Large white blood cells that turn into macrophages. They are often infected with *Chlamydophila pneumoniae*. Monocytes actually protect *C. pneumoniae* from some antibiotics.

Morning cortisol levels. The level of cortisol in the morning; a very unreliable indication of whether or not someone has hypercortisolism.

Mother Nature. A compact term for "the sum of all of the historical and evolutionary forces that make the world what it is and us what we are."

Myocardial infarction. *See* heart attack.

Necrosis of bone, aseptic. Death of bone not caused by an infection; a sign of hypercortisolism.

Nephropathy. Damage to the filters in the kidneys; a frequent complication of diabetes.

Neuropathy. A disease of the nervous system; a frequent complication of diabetes.

Nicotine. One of several insect poisons produced by tobacco plants.

Night-eating syndrome (NES). A powerful urge to eat at night. It has been linked to hypercortisolism.

Noninsulin-dependent diabetes mellitus (NIDDM). *See* Diabetes, type 2.

Obesity. An excessively high amount of body fat relative to lean body mass. Often defined as having a body mass index (BMI) of 30 or more.

Obesity, abdominal. A large amount of fat around the waist; includes visceral fat.

Obesity, diffuse. Subcutaneous fat diffused over much of the body.

Obesity, visceral. Excess fat around the organs contained by the abdominal muscles. This is the fat that is most dangerous to health; visceral fat is part of abdominal fat.

Opportunistic infection. An infection in an immunosuppressed person caused by an organism that does not usually trouble people with healthy immune systems. Opportunistic infections are common in patients with Cushing's syndrome and other forms of hypercortisolism.

Osteoarthritis. A form of arthritis in which the joints deteriorate; often exacerbated by hypercortisolism.

Osteonecrosis. Death of bone, especially at the hip joint, that leads to severe arthritis; often caused by hypercortisolism.

Osteoporosis. Loss of bone. Osteoporosis often causes vertebral fractures in people with hypercortisolism.

Pancreas. An organ that helps regulate glucose levels by producing more or less insulin. The pancreas also makes glucagon, a hormone that opposes insulin.

Pituitary gland. The "master gland" located behind the eyes. It regulates growth, metabolism, maturation, and reproduction. Also known as the *hypophysis.*

Plasma. The watery portion of the blood, in which the blood cells are suspended; the plasma contains minerals, nutrients, regulatory substances, gases, and proteins.

Platelets. Small, flat cellular fragments critical for clotting blood.

Polymerase chain reaction (PCR). A technique used to identify the DNA molecules of germs. PCR tests often indicate that a person's monocytes are infected with *Chlamydophila pneumoniae* even when antibody tests indicate that the person is not infected.

Potbelly syndrome. A dysmetabolic syndrome resembling the milder forms of Cushing's syndrome.

Primary cytokines. Interleukin-1 (IL-1), interleukin-6 (IL-6), and tumor necrosis factor-alpha (TNF-alpha). All three of the primary cytokines are pro-inflammatory, and all three stimulate cortisol production.

Protein. The main constituent of muscle cells. It is also needed to make hormones, enzymes, and antibodies. Proteins are made from amino acids.

Reaven's syndrome X (RSX). The mildest of the various dysmetabolic syndromes, and the first stage of potbelly syndrome.

Receptor. A protein usually found on the surface of a cell that recognizes and binds to cytokines and other chemical messengers.

Red blood cells. Cells that carry oxygen from the lungs to all of the other cells in the body.

Reference range. The "normal" range for a substance in the blood, saliva, or urine.

Septic shock. An often-fatal condition caused by an overwhelming infection. Cortisol levels are sometimes twentyfold higher than normal.

Signs. Markers for a disease that can be detected by special tests or instruments. Usually, they cannot be seen or felt by the patient. Compare with *symptom.*

Steatosis. The accumulation of fat in cells other than fat cells. A sign of hypercortisolism and insulin resistance.

Steroid psychosis. Depression and other mental problems caused by cortisol or cortisol-like medicines.

Stress and stressors. A *stress* is the effect that a *stressor* has on something. When a bus rolls across a bridge it pushes down on the bridge. The bus is the stressor and the "pushing down" is the stress. The bridge pushes up against the bus, and this "pushing up" is the bridge's response to stress. Different kinds of stressors can cause similar stresses. For examples, cars, buses, and trucks are different kinds of stressors, but they cause the same kind of "pushing down" stress. In ordinary speech, the word *stress* is often used to mean both *stress* and *stressor.*

Stress signals. Nerve or chemical signals that tell the hypothalamus something stressful is happening. The hypothalamus cannot distinguish between real and phony stress signals.

Stress spikes. Brief increases in stress levels.

Stress, phony. Stress caused by the imagination.

Stressor. *See* stress and stressors

Stressor, background. Any frequent or constant source of annoyance, anxiety, fear, infection, noise, pain, or worry.

Stroke. A "brain attack." Usually the result of chronic cerebrovascular disease. The blood vessels in the brain may become blocked (ischemic stroke). Sometimes, the blood vessels may burst (hemorrhagic stroke). Usually only one side of the body is affected.

Sucrose. Table sugar.

Supraoptimal. Above optimal. Usually means "slightly above optimal."

Symptom. An indication that a disease or disorder is present. It can be seen or felt by the patient. *See also* signs.

Syndrome. A recognizable set of signs and symptoms frequently found together. The signs and symptoms associated with a syndrome are usually assumed to arise from a common cause even if that common cause is not known.

Syndrome X. *See* Reaven's syndrome X.

Systolic blood pressure. The pressure that occurs each time the heart pushes blood into the arteries.

Triglyceride. The form in which fat cells store fatty acids. It is a combination of three fatty acid molecules and a glycerol molecule.

Tumor necrosis factor-alpha (TNF-alpha). Inflammatory cytokine, one of the primary cytokines that raise cortisol levels.

Tunica externa. The tough but very flexible outer layer of an artery made of small elastic fibers; also called the *adventitial* layer.

Tunica intima. Inner layer of an artery. This is the layer with the flat, delicate endothelial cells.

Tunica media. Middle layer of an artery. This is the layer with smooth muscles and baroreceptor nerves.

Ulcer. A lesion (or sore). Ulcers in the stomach are caused by a combination of stress and the bacterium *Helicobacter pylori.*

Ultrasound. The use of ultrasonic waves to produce an image of an internal body structure.

Vein. A blood vessel that carries blood toward the heart.

Virus. A noncellular germ that can only reproduce within a living host cell.

White blood cell. Immune cells that make up the first line of defense against infection and toxic agents; also called leukocytes. Monocytes and macrophages are white blood cells.

Index

About the Authors

Russell Farris spent thirty-eight years solving technical problems for the U.S. Navy and Air Force before retiring in 1994. He tracked Soviet submarines, directed the operations of missile-tracking ships at Cape Canaveral, and designed control systems for pilotless aircraft. After earning a degree in psychology from San Diego State University, Mr. Farris worked on artificial intelligence problems of interest to the Navy. After a heart attack in 1998, he began to apply his problem-solving skills to the prevention of obesity, diabetes, and heart disease.

Per Mårin, M.D., Ph.D., is a scientist, physician, and clinical instructor who has been studying obesity and type 2 diabetes for twenty years. His research has focused on finding ways to stop the progress of these diseases at the earliest possible stages, long before they contribute to morbidity or mortality. In 1991 he realized that hypersecretion of the stress hormone cortisol was the most plausible explanation for the wide range of symptoms associated with obesity and diabetes. Since then, most of his scientific publications have dealt with the effects of cortisol on weight and health. He is now overseeing clinical trials designed to identify medical treatments that will prevent type 2 diabetes and its complications. Dr. Mårin, who lives in Sweden, has been a guest lecturer at medical conferences throughout Europe and North America.

www.ingramcontent.com/pod-product-compliance
Lightning Source LLC
Jackson TN
JSHW011357130125
77033JS00023B/724

9781591200581